Methods in Molecular Biology

Series Editor
John M. Walker
School of Life and Medical Sciences
University of Hertfordshire, Hatfield
Hertfordshire, UK

For further volumes:
http://www.springer.com/series/7651

For over 35 years, biological scientists have come to rely on the research protocols and methodologies in the critically acclaimed *Methods in Molecular Biology* series. The series was the first to introduce the step-by-step protocols approach that has become the standard in all biomedical protocol publishing. Each protocol is provided in readily-reproducible step-by-step fashion, opening with an introductory overview, a list of the materials and reagents needed to complete the experiment, and followed by a detailed procedure that is supported with a helpful notes section offering tips and tricks of the trade as well as troubleshooting advice. These hallmark features were introduced by series editor Dr. John Walker and constitute the key ingredient in each and every volume of the *Methods in Molecular Biology* series. Tested and trusted, comprehensive and reliable, all protocols from the series are indexed in PubMed.

Cardiomyocytes

Methods and Protocols

Edited by

Dhananjie N. K. Chandrasekera and Rajesh Katare

Department of Physiology, HeartOtago, University of Otago, Dunedin, New Zealand

Humana Press

Editors
Dhananjie N. K. Chandrasekera
Department of Physiology, HeartOtago
University of Otago
Dunedin, New Zealand

Rajesh Katare
Department of Physiology, HeartOtago
University of Otago
Dunedin, New Zealand

ISSN 1064-3745 ISSN 1940-6029 (electronic)
Methods in Molecular Biology
ISBN 978-1-0716-4344-0 ISBN 978-1-0716-4342-6 (eBook)
https://doi.org/10.1007/978-1-0716-4342-6

This Humana imprint is published by the registered company Springer Science+Business Media, LLC, part of Springer Nature.
The registered company address is: 1 New York Plaza, New York, NY 10004, U.S.A.

Preface

Cardiomyocytes, the primary contractile cells of the heart, are pivotal to understanding cardiac function and the pathophysiology of various cardiovascular diseases. These specialized cells possess a unique architecture and functional capacity that underpin the heart's rhythmic contractions, orchestrating blood circulation throughout the body. In recent years, the study of cardiomyocytes has gained even greater prominence as researchers seek to explore their potential in regenerative therapies for heart disease and heart failure, leading causes of mortality worldwide.

The study of cardiomyocytes has evolved significantly over the past few decades, driven by advancements in technology and methodology. From initial explorations of their basic physiology to current studies unraveling their complex molecular mechanisms, cardiomyocyte research has continually expanded our knowledge. This book, *Cardiomyocytes: Methods and Protocols*, is a testament to these advancements. It combines diverse experimental approaches essential for researchers aiming to delve into the intricacies of cardiomyocyte biology and pathology.

This compilation is designed as a comprehensive resource that covers a broad range of experimental techniques, each presented with meticulous detail to ensure reproducibility and clarity. The book opens with fundamental protocols such as the isolation and culture of neonatal cardiomyocytes (Chap. 1) and the isolation of individual adult mouse cardiomyocytes (Chap. 2). These foundational techniques are crucial for establishing reliable in vitro models that allow for the detailed study of cardiomyocyte behavior under various physiological and pathological conditions. The book also covers specialized methodologies, such as isolating endothelial cells from the human internal mammary artery (Chap. 3), an essential technique for those studying the interaction between cardiomyocytes and the vasculature.

Moving beyond basic isolation methods, the book includes protocols for studying specific cellular processes and responses. For instance, Chaps. 4 and 5 explore functional assays, such as measuring mitochondrial membrane potential and lactate dehydrogenase activity in models of acute in vitro ischemia-reperfusion injury and inducing insulin resistance in vitro, both of which are critical to understanding metabolic changes that affect cardiomyocyte viability and function.

One of the strengths of this book is its inclusion of protocols that bridge in vitro studies with in vivo models, thereby providing a holistic approach to cardiomyocyte research. For example, Chap. 6 describes the preparation of human atrial trabeculae for functional studies of the human heart; Chap. 8 details the protocol for measuring vascular function using pressure myography. Chapter 9 presents the Langendorff isolated heart perfusion model for functional studies in mice. Such models are indispensable for exploring the effects of genetic modifications, pharmacological agents, and pathological conditions on heart and vascular function without interfering with other systems.

In addition to traditional methods, this book highlights cutting-edge techniques pushing the boundaries of cardiomyocyte research. Chapters 11 and 12, for example, delve into quantitative real-time PCR for circular RNA and small nucleolar RNA detection and analysis, a novel area of research that is uncovering new layers of gene regulation in cardiomyocytes. Chapter 14 introduces cationic liposome formulation by microfluidics for miRNA delivery, a state-of-the-art approach that holds promise for targeted gene therapy in cardiovascular diseases. The book also addresses the growing interest in cardiomyocyte interactions with other cell types and the extracellular environment. Chapter 10 describes the isolation of exosomes from pericardial fluids, offering a window into the complex communication networks between cardiomyocytes and surrounding cells.

Furthermore, the book addresses advanced techniques for studying cardiomyocyte function in vivo. Chapter 15 introduces methods for quantifying sympathetic nerve traffic to the heart, including electrophysiological recording of cardiac sympathetic nerve activity in rodent models. This protocol is invaluable for researchers interested in the neurocardiac axis and its role in cardiovascular diseases such as arrhythmias and heart failure. Additionally, Chap. 16 describes an ovine model of chronic heart failure induced by repeated coronary microembolization, which provides a large-animal model for studying the progression of heart failure and testing novel therapeutic approaches.

Throughout the book, readers will also find protocols for routine yet indispensable techniques such as western blotting (Chap. 13) and intracellular calcium measurement (Chap. 7). These chapters provide detailed step-by-step protocols that are invaluable for characterizing cardiomyocytes' molecular and electrophysiological properties under various experimental conditions.

The strength of this book lies not only in its comprehensive coverage of methods but also in the collective expertise and experience of its contributors. We are honored to have collaborated with leading scientists from various institutions worldwide, each of whom has shared their unique perspectives and specialized knowledge. Their dedication to advancing the field of cardiomyocyte research is evident in the clarity and precision of the protocols presented, making it a valuable resource for both novice and seasoned researchers in the field of cardiomyocyte research.

We hope this book will serve as a trusted guide for researchers exploring the complexities of cardiomyocyte biology and its implications for cardiovascular health and disease. Whether you are investigating the basic physiology of these remarkable cells or developing novel therapeutic strategies to combat heart disease, we trust that you will find these protocols informative and inspiring. We also hope that this book will foster collaboration and innovation within the scientific community, ultimately contributing to advancing cardiovascular research and improving human health.

Finally, we would like to express our deepest gratitude to our families, colleagues, and students, whose unwavering support has been instrumental in completing this project. Their encouragement and understanding have been a constant motivation throughout the editing process. We dedicate this book to all those who, through their curiosity and perseverance, seek to unlock the mysteries of the heart and contribute to improving human health.

With this preface, we invite you to embark on a journey through the fascinating world of cardiomyocyte research. May this book catalyze discoveries and innovations in cardiovascular science.

Dunedin, Otago, New Zealand ***Dhananjie N. K. Chandrasekera***
Rajesh Katare

Contents

Contributors

HAMISH M. AITKEN-BUCK • *Department of Physiology, HeartOtago, School of Biomedical Sciences, University of Otago, Dunedin, New Zealand*
ESTHER U. ASAMUDO • *Department of Pharmacology, University of California, Davis, CA, USA*
DEEPTHI ASHOK • *Division of Cardiology, Department of Medicine, Johns Hopkins University, Baltimore, MD, USA*
DONALD M. BERS • *Department of Pharmacology, University of California, Davis, CA, USA*
KYRA T. BINGHAM • *Department of Physiology, HeartOtago, School of Biomedical Sciences, University of Otago, Dunedin, New Zealand*
DHANANJIE N. K. CHANDRASEKERA • *Department of Cardiac Physiology, National Cerebral and Cardiovascular Center, Osaka, Japan*
TANYA R. CULLY • *Department of Physiology, HeartOtago, School of Biomedical Sciences, University of Otago, Dunedin, New Zealand*
OBIALUNANMA V. EBENEBE • *Bloomberg School of Public Health, Department of Environmental Health and Engineering, Johns Hopkins University, Baltimore, MD, USA*
MARTIN FRONIUS • *Department of Physiology, University of Otago, Dunedin, New Zealand; HeartOtago, University of Otago, Dunedin, New Zealand*
HALEY GARBUS • *Bloomberg School of Public Health, Department of Environmental Health and Engineering, Johns Hopkins University, Baltimore, MD, USA*
VENKATA NAGA SRIKANTH GARIKIPATI • *Aging + Cardiovascular Discovery Center, Department of Cardiovascular Sciences, Lewis Katz School of Medicine, Temple University, Philadelphia, PA, USA*
MADYSON O. HINTZ • *Department of Physiology and HeartOtago, School of Biomedical Sciences, University of Otago, Otago, New Zealand*
LARS JØRN JENSEN • *Department of Veterinary and Animal Sciences, Faculty of Health and Medical Sciences, University of Copenhagen, Copenhagen, Denmark*
PETER P. JONES • *Department of Physiology and HeartOtago, School of Biomedical Sciences, University of Otago, Otago, New Zealand*
YOSHIHIKO KAKINUMA • *Department of Bioregulatory Science, Nippon Medical School, Tokyo, Japan*
REGIS R. LAMBERTS • *Department of Physiology, HeartOtago, School of Biomedical Sciences, University of Otago, Dunedin, New Zealand*
HEIDY K. LATCHMAN • *School of Agriculture, Biomedicine and Environment, La Trobe University, Melbourne, VIC, Australia*
TIFFANY LEE • *Aging + Cardiovascular Discovery Center, Department of Cardiovascular Sciences, Lewis Katz School of Medicine, Temple University, Philadelphia, PA, USA*
JAMES A. LOEHR • *Department of Physiology, HeartOtago, School of Biomedical Sciences, University of Otago, Dunedin, New Zealand*
FIONA MCDONALD • *Department of Physiology, University of Otago, Dunedin, New Zealand*
ROBYN M. MURPHY • *School of Agriculture, Biomedicine and Environment, La Trobe University, Melbourne, VIC, Australia*
YANN HUEY NG • *Charles Perkins Centre, School of Medical Sciences, Faculty of Medicine and Health, The University of Sydney, Sydney, NSW, Australia*

MRIDULA PACHEN • *Manaaki Manawa – The Centre for Heart Research and the Department of Physiology, University of Auckland, Auckland, New Zealand*
PUJA PAUDEL • *Department of Physiology, University of Otago, Dunedin, New Zealand; HeartOtago, University of Otago, Dunedin, New Zealand*
AMELIA S. POWER • *Department of Physiology, University of Auckland, Auckland, New Zealand*
AMIT KUMAR RAI • *Aging + Cardiovascular Discovery Center, Department of Cardiovascular Sciences, Lewis Katz School of Medicine, Temple University, Philadelphia, PA, USA*
ROHIT RAMCHANDRA • *Manaaki Manawa – The Centre for Heart Research and the Department of Physiology, University of Auckland, Auckland, New Zealand; Department of Physiology, Faculty of Medical and Health Sciences, University of Auckland, Auckland, New Zealand*
MATTHEW REILY-BELL • *Department of Physiology and School of Pharmacy, Division of Health Sciences, University of Otago, Dunedin, New Zealand*
ENG LENG SAW • *Whitaker Cardiovascular Institute, Boston University Chobanian & Avedisian School of Medicine, Boston, MA, USA*
DARYL O. SCHWENKE • *Department of Physiology, School of Biomedical Science, University of Otago, Dunedin, New Zealand*
RISHI SHAH • *Department of Physiology and School of Pharmacy, Division of Health Sciences, University of Otago, Dunedin, New Zealand*
MARIE-LOUISE WARD • *Department of Physiology, University of Auckland, Auckland, New Zealand*
UTE ZELLHUBER-MCMILLAN • *Department of Physiology and HeartOtago, School of Biomedical Sciences, University of Otago, Otago, New Zealand*

Chapter 1

Isolating and Culturing Neonatal Cardiomyocytes

Yoshihiko Kakinuma

Abstract

Isolation of primary cardiomyocytes can be performed for studies from fetuses and neonates. Compared with rat neonatal cardiomyocytes, mouse neonatal cardiomyocytes are sensitive to enzyme digestion. Therefore, they need to optimize a concentration of collagenase and a time point to collect the heart after birth. In addition, neonatal cardiomyocytes have unique characteristics to be recognized although the preparation steps are not complicated. Therefore, depending on a researcher's interest and aim, they consider which sources of cardiomyocytes are suitable and convenient, for example, a rat or mouse, as well as a fetus and neonate.

Key words Mouse, Rat, Primary culture, Cardiomyocyte, Collagenase, Differential adhesion

1 Introduction

Cultured cardiomyocytes, especially from rats and mice, have been used in many studies, to understand their responses to drugs, genetic modulations, or stressors. Furthermore, depending on the goals and objectives of the study, adult or neonatal cardiomyocytes are selected. Although iPS-derived cardiomyocytes are also used for research, they take longer to obtain differentiated cardiomyocytes, and there is a risk of contamination by other cell types, as well as difficulty in regulating differentiation levels.

When using cultured cardiomyocytes, it is essential to consider which type of cardiomyocytes are the most useful for each experiment in terms of their characteristics and limitations [1, 2].

Primary cultured cardiomyocytes, from neonates or adults, are usually obtained by enzyme digestion and cultured in glucose-rich culture medium [2]. Therefore, this is a completely different environment for cultured cardiomyocytes in vitro compared to that for cardiomyocytes in vivo. In terms of energy metabolism, adult cardiomyocytes in the whole body predominantly utilize fatty acids to synthesize ATP more efficiently than glucose. However, in cultured adult cardiomyocytes, their preference for fatty acid may be

Dhananjie N. K. Chandrasekera and Rajesh Katare (eds.), *Cardiomyocytes: Methods and Protocols*, Methods in Molecular Biology, vol. 2894, https://doi.org/10.1007/978-1-0716-4342-6_1,

suppressed and shifted to glucose. On the other hand, neonatal cardiomyocytes in vivo initially rely on glucose and then gradually shift to fatty acids to synthesize more ATP. Based on the efficient bidirectional shift in energy metabolism, which is equipped by cardiomyocytes, neonatal cardiomyocytes in vitro may also switch from fatty acids to glucose under specific culture conditions such as glucose-rich culture medium or loss of physiological massive contraction. However, this may be a pathological state (a glucose-dependent state) and may not observed in healthy cardiomyocytes in vivo (a fatty acid-dependent state) [3]. In this aspect, they need to consider and evaluate the influence of in vitro environment on results they obtain.

Additionally, adult mouse cardiomyocytes usually show a rod-shaped appearance after enzyme digestion. As a result, the digested ends of adult cardiomyocytes lose their connection with neighboring cardiomyocytes. Therefore, the adult cardiomyocytes gradually show a round morphology and cause disorganization of muscle fibers, leading to loss of its original structure during the progression of culture. Thus, a culture duration may be limited in adult mouse cardiomyocytes, compared with neonatal mouse cardiomyocytes. This is a limitation of using cultured adult mouse cardiomyocytes [4]. In contrast, rat adult cardiomyocytes can be cultured for more prolonged time period than mouse adult cardiomyocytes, and this is an advantage over adult mouse cardiomyocytes.

Furthermore, when isolating cardiomyocytes from a mouse, it is easier to obtain fetal cardiomyocytes at full term rather than neonatal cardiomyocytes post-delivery day 1, as neonatal cardiomyocytes are more prone to cell death probably due to higher susceptibility to cell damage during digestion. This is clearly in contrast to rat cardiomyocytes. When using mouse neonates, they need to optimize specifically when the hearts are excised even during post-delivery day 1 [5, 6]. In contrast, different from mouse neonates, rat neonatal hearts can be used for isolation until post-deliver day 3. Based on this, rat neonatal cardiomyocytes can be prepared more easily with more yield. This is another limitation of mouse neonatal cardiomyocytes. Although adequate neonatal cardiomyocytes can be obtained by our protocol, more vital fetal cardiomyocytes can be obtained from full-term fetuses; however, the cells are smaller in fetal cardiomyocytes than in neonatal cardiomyocytes. In addition, rat neonatal cardiomyocytes continued beating for a more prolonged duration than mouse cardiomyocytes. Despite the several advantages, many genetically modified models are available in mice, and this prompts us to adapt the isolation protocol for mouse neonatal cardiomyocytes, which are more efficient to be transfected. Before establishing this method, it is important to optimize which sources, fetuses, or neonates, is better for your study.

2 Materials

2.1 Tissue Collection

1. Digestion buffer:30 mM HEPES, 121 mM NaCl, 4 mM dextrose, 2 mM KCl, 1 mM KH_2PO_4, pH 7.6, filtrated with 0.2 μm filter.
2. Collagenase solution: collagenase types 2 and 4 (1:1).

A final total collagenase concentration is set 0.1% in total 10 mL digestion buffer. Therefore, 5 mg each collagenase (total 10 mg) in 10 mL digestion buffer.

Collagenase types 2 and 4: Worthington Biochemical Corporation (Lakewood, NJ, USA) #LS004176, LS004186, respectively

3. 48-well plate.
4. 10 cm culture dish.
5. Cell strainer (70 μm).
6. 50 mL and 15 mL tubes
7. Incubator bath (37 °C).

2.2 Cell Culture

1. DMEM F-12 complete medium, 2% FBS.
2. DMEM F-12 complete medium, 5% FBS, ×100 antibiotic–antimycotic solution, and ×100 insulin-transferrin-selenate (ITS)-G supplement.
3. DMEM F-12 complete medium, 2% FBS, ×100 antibiotic–antimycotic solution, and ×100 insulin-transferrin-selenate (ITS)-G supplement.
4. DMEM F-12 complete medium, 1% FBS, ×100 antibiotic–antimycotic solution, and ×100 insulin-transferrin-selenate (ITS)-G supplement.
5. 10 μg/mL human fibronectin solution: For usage, stock 1 mg/mL human fibronectin solution is diluted to ×100 to a 10 μg/mL working solution with 1 × PBS (−).

3 Methods

1. Mate male and female mice. The next day, check for a vaginal plug in the female mouse.
2. Starting from checking the plug (day 1), observe the progression of pregnancy from day 1 to day 21.
3. When a female pregnant mouse is close to delivering babies, usually on day 20 or 21, it is euthanized by cervical dislocation. The fetuses are removed from the uterus and placed in a 10 cm culture dish, which is kept on ice.

4. A fetal neck is cut using scissors and the cross section of the neck is then placed on a Kim towel to remove any residual blood. This procedure allows for easy identification of the fetal heart.
5. When using a stereomicroscope to perform a dissection, carefully insert scissors at the cross section of the trunk. Cut only the middle of the anterior thoracic wall, which is the middle of the sternum, using scissors. It is important to be cautious and avoid harming the heart.
6. The heart is visible, under the stereomicroscope, with two chambers containing residual blood. In contrast, the thymus and lungs surrounding the heart do not contain adequate blood. The different appearance allows us to precisely detect the heart. Therefore, it is essential to completely remove the residual blood using a Kim towel.
7. Excise hearts. Usually, eight fetal hearts are obtained from a pregnant female mouse. They are washed multiple times in a digestion buffer (without collagenase). Remove fibrous tissue and atria from the heart using micro-scissors.
8. Then, all the hearts are transferred to a 10 mL solution of 0.1% collagenase and incubated at 37 °C for 15 min with agitation (*see* **Note 1**). Fifteen minutes later, hearts are pipetted several times, and digestion continues for an additional 15 min.
9. After the next 15 min (a total of 30 min after the start of digestion), the supernatant is transferred into a new 50 mL tube and 1 mL of FBS is added to it.
10. The residual tissue left from no. 9, which can be seen at the bottom of the tube, is again treated with a new 0.1% collagenase solution (5 mL) at 37 °C for 15 min and then pipetted several times. Digestion is continued for another 15 min (*see* **Note 1**).
11. After 60 min of incubation, the second supernatant is transferred again to the new 50 mL tube to obtain 20 mL digested heart. The digested cardiomyocytes are centrifuges at 1000 rpm, 4 °C for 4 min and resuspended in 4 mL of the digestion buffer.
12. Then, the mixed supernatant is poured to a cell strainer (70 μm).
13. Centrifuge it at 1000 rpm, 4 °C for 4 min. Then the pellet is again resuspended in 4 mL of the digestion buffer and recentrifuged likewise.
14. The pellet is resuspended in 10 mL of DMEM/F12 culture medium with 2% FBS.

15. A multiwell plate is coated with fibronectin (10 μg/mL), which is diluted ×100 times from 1 mg/mL by 1 × PBS (−), and kept at 37 °C for more than 30 min (*see* **Note 2**).
16. To exclude extra-cardiomyocytes, particularly fibroblasts, the cardiomyocytes are subjected to differential adhesion using a 10 cm culture dish. This is an important step for exclusion of extra-cardiomyocytes, especially fibroblasts. The adhesion duration for extra-cardiomyocytes should be optimized, depending on a condition of digestion in cardiomyocytes as well as fibroblasts. Fibroblasts tend to attach more rapidly to a culture dish compared to cardiomyocytes. Observe under a microscope to check how many cells are attached. Usually, a duration of less than 5 min is required.
17. After the differential adhesion, the culture dish is gently agitated, and the supernatant is collected, and centrifuged at 1000 rpm at room temperature for 2 min.
18. The cardiomyocyte pellet is then resuspended in 2 mL of DMEM F-12 culture medium including 5% FBS, 1 × ITS, and antibiotics.
19. The cell count is usually around or below 1×10^6 cells in total from the 8–10 fetuses.
20. In a 48-well plate, 1.0×10^5 cells can be inoculated in each well on day 0.
21. After several hours, each cardiomyocyte attaches to the bottom of the dish and appears in a rhomboid or rod shape. If the isolation of cardiomyocytes is successful, some cardiomyocytes start to beat separately several hours after adhesion.
22. On day 2 after inoculation, the concentration of FBS alone is changed from 5% to 2% in the culture medium. Separated cardiomyocytes start to communicate with each other and gradually beat simultaneously. Finally, on day 4 or thereafter, a FBS concentration can be decreased to 1%, while the other contents remain the same, i.e., DMEM F-12 with 1 × ITS and antibiotics. Depending on a study protocol, the final FBS concentration may be varied. Usually, in the case of adequate cell number, cardiomyocytes beat synchronously on a culture dish after day 5–6.

4 Notes

1. Following several experiences with good yield of mouse cardiomyocytes, when the final yield of mouse cardiomyocytes abruptly becomes very low, the quality of collagenase should be considered. In that case, new collagenase should be purchased. In addition, if the yield of cardiomyocytes is not

improved, the concentration of a collagenase mixture may be relatively higher. Therefore, it should be modified to be decreased to less than 0.1%. Usually, a 0.1% collagenase mixture works well, however, more than 0.1% is usually harmful, especially for mouse neonatal hearts.

2. In this protocol, we use fibronectin to coat culture dishes. When cardiomyocytes are cultured on fibronectin, they become more flattened, resulting in an increase in their size, i.e., hypertrophy. This makes it easier to observe mouse cardiomyocytes in detail. However, when it is not necessary, gelatin can be used instead. The recommended concentration is 0.1%; however, it can be adjusted as per requirement.

References

1. Harary I, Farley B (1960) In vitro studies of single isolated beating heart cells. Science 131: 1674–1675. https://doi.org/10.1126/science.131.3414.1674
2. Ehler E, Moore-Morris T, Lange S (2013) Isolation and culture of neonatal mouse cardiomyocytes. J Vis Exp 79:50154. https://doi.org/10.3791/50154
3. Eppenberger HM, Hertig C, Eppenberger-Eberhardt M (1994) Adult rat cardiomyocytes in culture a model system to study the plasticity of the differentiated cardiac phenotype at the molecular and cellular levels. Trends Cardiovasc Med 4:187–193. https://doi.org/10.1016/1050-1738(94)90056-6
4. Judd J, Lovas J, Huang NG (2016) Isolation, culture and transduction of adult mouse Cardiomyocytes. J Vis Exp 114:54012. https://doi.org/10.3791/54012
5. Nicks AM, Holman SR, Chan AY, Tsang M, Young PE, Humphreys DT, Naqvi N, Husain A, Li M, Smith NJ, Iismaa SE, Robert M (2022) Graham standardised method for cardiomyocyte isolation and purification from individual murine neonatal, infant, and adult hearts. J Mol Cell Cardiol 170:47–59. https://doi.org/10.1016/j.yjmcc.2022.05.012
6. Kakinuma Y, Tsuda M, Okazaki K, Akiyama T, Arikawa M, Noguchi T, Sato T (2013) Heart-specific overexpression of choline acetyltransferase gene protects murine heart against ischemia through hypoxia-inducible factor-1α-related defense mechanisms. J Am Heart Assoc 2: e004887. https://doi.org/10.1161/JAHA.112.004887

Chapter 2

Simple Method to Isolate Individual Mouse Cardiomyocytes Using Enzymatic Digestion via Retrograde Perfusion

Madyson O. Hintz, Ute Zellhuber-McMillan, and Peter P. Jones

Abstract

Isolated single cardiomyocytes are commonly used to understand fundamental cardiac cell physiology and cell signaling at the molecular level. The protocol to isolate cardiomyocytes is under continual optimization between laboratories, despite being conducted for many years. The delicate nature of these cells coinciding with laboratory equipment variations can make the consistency of isolation challenging. The protocol described here presents a simple method to routinely isolate high-quality cardiomyocytes using Langendorff perfusion. This method provides cells well suited for analysis of physiological cellular calcium handling and spontaneous calcium release.

Key words Cardiomyocytes, Cell isolation, Langendorff, Cardiac physiology

1 Introduction

The method of isolating adult murine cardiomyocytes has been conducted for almost a half century, resulting in a mass of publications [1–3]. Despite the large number of publications available, compared to other species, the isolation of adult mouse cardiomyocytes remains challenging. The complexity of the technique and sensitive nature of the cells means even small errors can affect the success of the isolation. Most methods use a combination of mechanical dissociation and enzymatic digestion processes to break down the extracellular matrix between adjacent cells. However, there remains a delicate balance between ensuring sufficient dissociation of cells to obtain a usable yield and excessive digestion that disrupts the cell membrane, compromising cardiomyocyte integrity [4].

There are two main protocols for cardiomyocyte isolation. The least technically challenging is the bulk, or chunk, digestion method. This simplistic approach involves gross dissection of the

Dhananjie N. K. Chandrasekera and Rajesh Katare (eds.), *Cardiomyocytes: Methods and Protocols*, Methods in Molecular Biology, vol. 2894, https://doi.org/10.1007/978-1-0716-4342-6_2,

heart into small (1 mm^3) pieces before enzymatic digestion and trituration of the tissue [5]. Although this technique can produce viable cardiomyocytes, the yield is typically low compared to other methods. Despite the relatively small size of the tissue pieces, there is still variable exposure of the tissue to the enzymes resulting in the outer tissue typically being over-digested (poor membrane integrity) and the inner tissue being under-digested (little to no breakdown of extracellular matrix) [6]. Consequently, this technique is typically reserved for tissue that cannot be dissociated using a perfusion technique (see below). A common use of chunk digestions is the isolation of cardiomyocytes from human tissue where due to the nature of the sample, often a biopsy or small excision, perfusion is not possible.

Where possible, the favored method of cardiomyocyte isolation is perfusion-based digestion. In the case of rodent hearts, this is achieved using a Langendorff apparatus. The technique exploits the coronary vasculature of the heart to deliver solutions deep into the tissue ensuring a similar exposure of all cells to the enzymes. Once the extracellular matrix is sufficiently degraded, trituration is then used to liberate individual cells. However, despite the more consistent exposure of cardiomyocytes to the enzyme, a successful isolation is highly dependent on the enzyme type, batch, and duration of digestion.

To minimize variation and increase success standardized protocols have been developed which utilize specially formulated enzyme blends (e.g., Liberase, Merck, MO, USA). While these provide high levels of consistency, they do so at a high cost, making using such reagents prohibitively expensive for many groups. Therefore, it is common that laboratories make their own blend of enzymes. While this can result in comparable success to those using standardized blends, careful optimization must occur between batches, necessitating greater experimenter experience to determine when optimal digestion has taken place.

There are several enzyme blends described by different groups; however, the protocol described below only uses collagenase type II, reducing cost and complexity (Worthington Biochemical Corporation, NJ, USA). This enzyme is favored for heart tissue digestion due to its high protease activity, more specifically clostripain, and is commonly used in the field. In addition to enzyme choice and concentration, other parameters that can impact digestion are temperature, calcium concentration, and heart size. Each of which must be considered to optimize cell isolation within an individual laboratory.

Despite the challenges of isolation, single cardiomyocytes have proven to be invaluable in the study of heart function at a cellular and molecular level. Acute harvesting of cardiomyocytes allows many in vivo characteristics to be maintained. Despite no longer being bound to adjacent cells, single cells are frequently used to study intrinsic mechanisms such as force-length relationships [7, 8] and calcium handling [9] and how this may be altered with interventions such as pharmaceuticals, genetic mutations, or adaptions in cardiac function and disease. With developing technologies and intracellular signaling indicators, an ever-increasing range of intracellular events can be assessed.

While Langendorff isolation of cardiomyocytes is possible for all animals, it is most often used with rodents, typically mice and rats. Despite significant differences to larger mammalian hearts [10], the rapid life cycle and aging and ease of genetic manipulation make these the models of choice. Literature most commonly uses mice of 8–12 weeks of age [11] as they represent an adult heart and is an age where the success of isolation is highest. Using younger or older animals is more challenging due to more difficult cannulation and cardiomyocytes more prone to damage during isolation, respectively [12].

Therefore, the methodology below is optimized for collagenase type II-based isolation of murine cardiomyocytes isolated from 8–12-week-old animals. The method is simple and cost-effective while providing a high yield of ventricular cells suitable for calcium imaging and studying contractile function.

2 Materials

2.1 Langendorff Apparatus (See Note 1, Fig. 1)

1. Two 75 mL reservoirs.
2. Peroxide silicone tubing (ID: 2.8 mm).
3. Three-way valve.
4. Water jackets heated by a water bath circulator.
5. O_2 supply to each reservoir via bubblers.
6. A 20 gauge blunt tip cannula with a circumferential notch approximately 1.5 mm from the end.

2.2 Buffers (See Note 2)

1. Ca^{2+}-free Krebs-Ringer-HEPES (KRH) buffer: NaCl 125 mM, KCL 5 mM, HEPES 5 mM, $MgCl_2$ 1.2 mM, glucose 6 mM. pH 7.4.
2. Ca^{2+}- Krebs-Ringer-HEPES (KRH) buffers made by adding $CaCl_2$ to the buffer above: Different concentrations of Ca^{2+} are made according to Table 1.
3. Digestion buffer: collagenase type II (30 mg) dissolved in 30 mL of 0.125 mM Ca^{2+}-KRH (provides a 1 mg/mL concentration).
4. Collagenase Type II (*see* **Note 3** and Table 2).

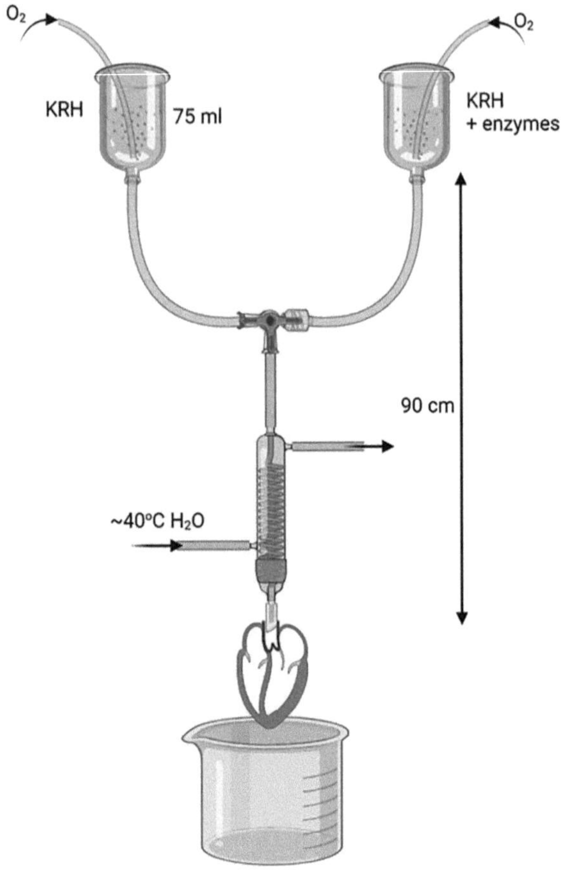

Fig. 1 Schematic of Langendorff perfusion apparatus. Components not drawn to scale. (KRH, Krebs-Ringer-HEPES)

Table 1
Ca^{2+}-Krebs-Ringer-HEPES (KRH) buffers made by adding $CaCl_2$ to the buffer

Ca^{2+}-KRH buffer	1 mM Ca^{2+}	0.1 mM Ca^{2+}	0.125 mM Ca^{2+}
$CaCl_2$ (2 M)	25 μL	–	–
KRH	50 mL	45 mL	26.25 mL
1 mM Ca^{2+}-KRH	–	5 mL	3.75 mL
Total volume	50 mL	50 mL	30 mL

2.3 Dissection Tools

1. Fine scissors ToughCut straight.
2. Extra-fine Graefe forceps (×2).
3. Tissue forceps 1 × 2 teeth.
4. Westcott spring scissors slightly curved.

Table 2
Properties of collagenase type II shown to result in a high yield of cells using this protocol. u/mg dw = units per mg of dry weight. One unit liberates 1 μmole L-leucine from collagen in 5 h at 37.5 °C, pH 7.5

Parameter	Result
u/mg dw	310
u/mg dw caseinase	585
u/mg dw clostripain	5.75
u/mg dw tryptic	0.6
Endotoxin EU/mg dw	37.9
A280nm @ 1 mg/mL	1.89

5. Dumont #5/45 forceps (×2).
6. Dissection tray.
7. 15 mL conical tubes (×5).
8. 3 mL graduated transfer pipettes (×4).
9. 50 mL beaker (×2).
10. Braided silk suture 3–0.
11. Petri dish 100 × 20 mm.
12. 70 mL weight boat.
13. Nylon mesh 250 um.

3 Methods

3.1 Experimental Setup

1. On the day of use, wash the entire Langendorff apparatus with 70% ethanol by filling both 75 mL reservoirs and allowing it to run through all the tubing.
2. Remove residual ethanol using MilliQ H_2O.
3. Rinse with 150 mL of Ca^{2+}-free KRH buffer twice.
4. Turn on circulating water bath (heated water jacket) during these washes to allow the water to reach 40 °C.
5. Fill the left reservoir and tubing with Ca^{2+}-free KRH buffer.
6. Remove bubbles from the apparatus by flicking the tubing and flushing solution behind them to send the bubbles toward the bubble trap (*see* **Note 4**).
7. Reset the bubble trap as part of this process. To the right reservoir, add half of the 0.125 mM Ca^{2+}-KRH (15 mL).
8. Oxygenate these solutions with 100% O_2 while preparing the animal (*see* Subheading 3.2) and keep the O_2 flowing for the

entirety of the experiment. O_2 flow rate should result in gentle bubbling of the solution.

9. Incubate the 0.1 mM and remaining half of 0.125 mM Ca^{2+}-KRH solution in 40 °C water bath ready for later use (*see* Subheading 3.4.1).

3.2 Animal Preparation

1. C57BL/6 mice were used in this protocol at 8–12 weeks of age. All manipulations were approved by the University of Otago Animal Ethics Committee (AUP-19-43).
2. Rapidly anesthetize mouse using isoflurane (5% at 0.6 L/min) by placing in an induction box. We find that this method of anesthesia results in less stress on the animal.
3. Confirm the animal is in a surgical plane of anesthesia by the loss of the pedal withdrawal reflex upon pinching the toes of the hind leg.
4. Perform secondary confirmation using the corneal reflex by gently touching the eye with forceps. Upon confirmation of anesthesia, perform a cervical dislocation to euthanize the mouse.
5. Place the mouse in a supine position and using toothed forceps pull the xiphoid process of the sternum up and, using the fine scissors ToughCut straight, make an incision through the skin and abdominal wall.
6. Extend the incision down either side of the rib cage following the lower aspect of the ribs, making sure not to damage any underlying structures.
7. While still holding the sternum, use the scissors to carefully cut the diaphragm starting from each side working inward to the sternum.
8. Cut the heart's fibrous pericardial attachment to the diaphragm. It is very important here not to damage the heart; you can switch to using blunt-ended scissors or blunt-tipped forceps if you prefer.
9. Cut up through each side of the rib cage until you can easily reflect it back to expose the thoracic cavity.
10. Pull away any attachments of the thymus, cutting the thymus back if it obscures the atria.

3.3 Heart Excision and Cannulation

1. Using curved forceps, reach underneath the heart from the apex until the forceps lie slightly superior to the atria.
2. With the heart resting on the curve of the forceps, lift the heart to expose the major vessels. In one motion, cut the major vessels ~2 mm above the atria and lift the heart out.
3. Ensure to avoid piercing the atria as this will impact heart perfusion.

4. Aim to retain ~2 mm of aorta, too long and the aorta is hard to spot quickly as it is likely to collapse on itself. Too short and the aorta will be hard to cannulate and increases the likelihood of the cannula damaging or protruding through the aortic valve.
5. Immediately place the heart in the petri dish with ice-cold (~4 °C) Ca^{2+}-free KRH. This will arrest the heart.
6. Wash remnants of blood by very gently pressing on the chambers using the back of the forceps to clear them.
7. Using two pairs of fine-tip forceps, transfer the heart to the cannula on the Langendorff apparatus.
8. Use one of the fine-tip forceps to hold the aorta, using the other fine-tip forceps to gently stretch and open the aorta up over the cannula, above the aortic valve. Care must be taken to ensure the cannula only just enters the aorta to avoid penetrating and damaging the aortic valve.
9. Secure the aorta to the cannula with a braided silk tie. The suture should sit in the notch of the blunt-ended cannula (*see* **Note 5**).
10. To aid in securing the aorta, it is helpful to form a loop in the braided tie and slide over the cannula before mounting the heart.
11. Once mounted, the aorta will seal against the cannula, giving time for the loop to be lowered and tied around the aorta.
12. Perfuse the heart with Ca^{2+}-free KRH buffer until the perfusate runs clear of blood. Ensure there is no leakage from the cannulation.
13. The time from excision to cannulation and initial perfusion should be completed <1 min. Completing this quickly requires practice. Typically, it is recommended that new users practice canulating and then removing a heart repeatedly until this timing can be achieved before continuing the process.

3.4 Cell Isolation

3.4.1 Enzymatic Digestion

1. Once the perfusate is clear of blood, add the remaining 0.125 mM Ca^{2+}-KRH (15 mL) from the water bath to a beaker containing the 30 mg of collagenase.
2. Once dissolved, add to the reservoir containing the other 15 mL of 0.125 mM Ca^{2+}-KRH. Adding the solution to the enzyme at this point means the enzyme is not wasted should cannulation fail to be completed quickly.
3. Using the three-way valve, start perfusing the heart with the 0.125 mM Ca^{2+}-KRH collagenase solution.
4. The clearing of blood and switching to the enzyme-containing solution should take no longer than 3 min as to avoid the effects of the calcium paradox [13].

5. At this stage, the heart should appear pink without poorly perfused zones (darker or gray regions). If there are any noticeable poorly perfused zones (largely due to clots within the coronary arteries), a 27 G needle can be used to pierce the vasculature to remove the clot and to improve tissue perfusion (*see* **Note 6**).
6. As the enzymatic digestion proceeds, the heart should begin to look glassy/translucent and slightly enlarged.
7. The perfusate drops will become "droopy" or viscous in appearance and larger in size. The drip rate should also increase twofold from the initial rate.
8. The time it takes to reach optimal digestion is enzyme batch dependent, but if using enzyme with characteristics like those in Table 2, it should take ~8–12 min.
9. Before vessel integrity is completely lost and the tissue changes from pink to gray or white, stop perfusion with digestion buffer. *See* Fig. 2 for examples of how the heart appearance changes during the digestion process.
10. It is important to have good lighting to see these changes clearly. Cut the heart to remove ventricles using the fine scissors.
11. Place the ventricles into 10 mL of 0.1 mM Ca^{2+}-KRH.
12. The atria should be more translucent and easily distinguishable from the ventricles.
13. If unclear, cut the bottom three-fourths of the heart tissue down, below the atrial lobes (*see* **Note 7**).
14. Further dissection into left and right ventricles can be performed at this stage if desired.

3.4.2 Mechanical Dissociation

1. Mince the ventricles using the fine scissors ToughCut straight until tissue is approximately 1–2 mm^3 in size and decant the supernatant into a 15 mL tube.
2. Remove any coagulated blood from the tissue. This step removes the bulk of the collagenase solution and other unwanted matter such as fibrous tissue and endothelial or red blood cells.
3. Add another 10 mL of 0.1 mM Ca^{2+}-KRH to the tissue. Use a wide-bore transfer pipette to gently triturate the tissue using suction and forced expulsion. If the tissue exerts too much resistance to being sucked into the pipette, the tissue chunks are too large and should be minced further (*see* **Note 8**). Start by pipetting solution onto the tissue to break them down. Forcing large pieces of tissue into the pipette can damage the cells.

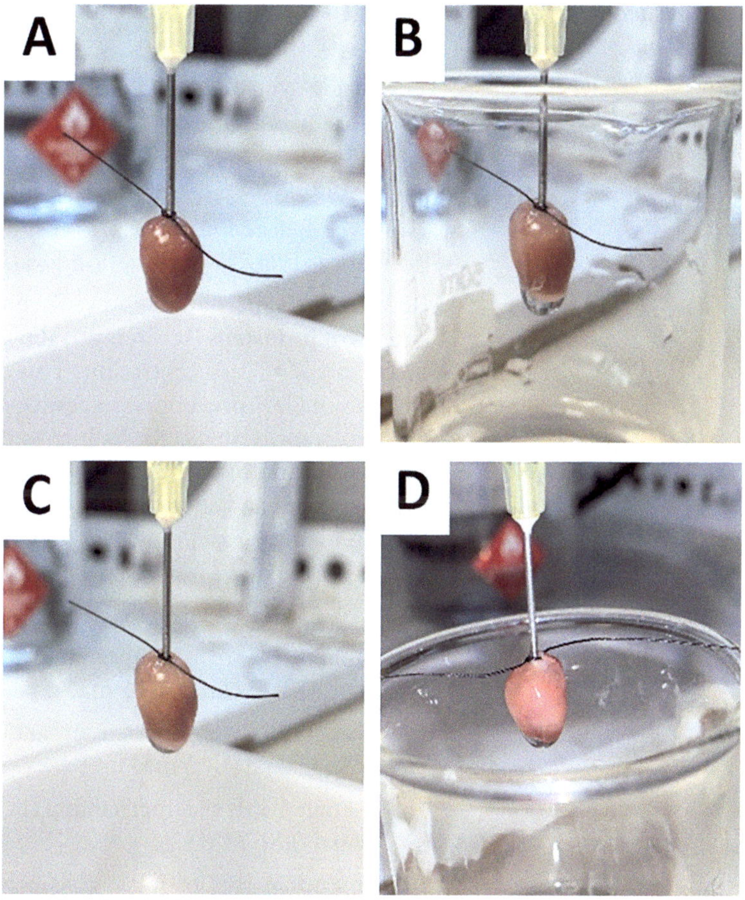

Fig. 2 Mouse heart attached to the blunt-tip cannula. (**a**) Before enzymatic digestion. (**b**) During enzymatic digestion. Note the color change and glassier appearance. (**c**) Over-digested heart, note its pale/gray appearance. (**d**) Another over-digested heart, note here the white zones near the apex

4. Once the tissue chunks are small enough, suck the tissue up into the pipette and expel back onto the bottom of the beaker.
5. When the supernatant is cloudy/opaque, and most visible chunks have been dissociated, decant into another 15 mL tube.
6. During titration, the tissue should break down becoming a stringlike consistency without too much resistance (*see* **Note 9**).
7. Repeat this step a further three times.
8. On the final supernatant decantation, use 250 μm nylon mesh to filter cells from remaining tissue chunks.
9. In total, five tubes of supernatant are collected, each with approximately 10 mL.

3.5 Calcium Restoration/Reintroduction and Cell Sedimentation

1. Allow 10 min for the healthy cardiomyocytes to settle in the bottom of the 15 mL tube.
2. The dead/over-digested cells and non-myocytes will not precipitate and largely remain within the supernatant. At this point, the cardiomyocytes are partially depleted of Ca^{2+}; this preserves the cell's metabolic function.
3. However, before use, the Ca^{2+} must be restored slowly to study normal cardiomyocyte function [14].
4. Remove the supernatant and replace with 1 mM Ca^{2+}-KRH in a series of four steps (see below), allowing 10 min between each increase in Ca^{2+} concentration. This ensures a gradual reintroduction of Ca^{2+} preventing excessive cell damage and produces Ca^{2+}-tolerant, viable cells. Failure to do this gradually results in the Ca^{2+} paradox, whereby rapid reintroduction of Ca^{2+} to isolated cells can cause morphological changes and damage to the sarcolemma [13].
   (i) Retain 3.5 mL of supernatant, and add 0.5 mL of 1 mM Ca^{2+}-KRH (final 0.25 mM).
   (ii) Retain 3.0 mL of supernatant, and add 1 mL of 1 mM Ca^{2+}-KRH (final 0.44 mM).
   (iii) Retain 2 mL of supernatant, and add 1 mL of 1 mM Ca^{2+}-KRH (final 0.72 mM).
   (iv) Retain 1 mL of supernatant, and add 1 mL of Ca^{2+}-KRH (final 0.86 mM).
5. At the end of this process, cells are suspended in 0.86 mM Ca^{2+}-KRH. Under these conditions, cells are typically stable for several hours at room temperature.

3.6 Cell Yield and Viability

High-quality cells can now be identified using a visual checklist.

1. Use a pipette to transfer a small amount from each cardiomyocyte precipitate to a slide to inspect their cellular viability.
2. Viable cardiomyocytes will be rod-shaped with clear striations and defined edges (Fig. 3). They will contain no membrane blebs and granulations and have no spontaneous contractility. These cells should be in high abundance (*see* **Note 10**).

3.7 Cleaning Apparatus

To avoid contamination post-experiment, the Langendorff apparatus is flushed three times with hot (recently boiled) MilliQ H_2O before a final wash with 70% ethanol.

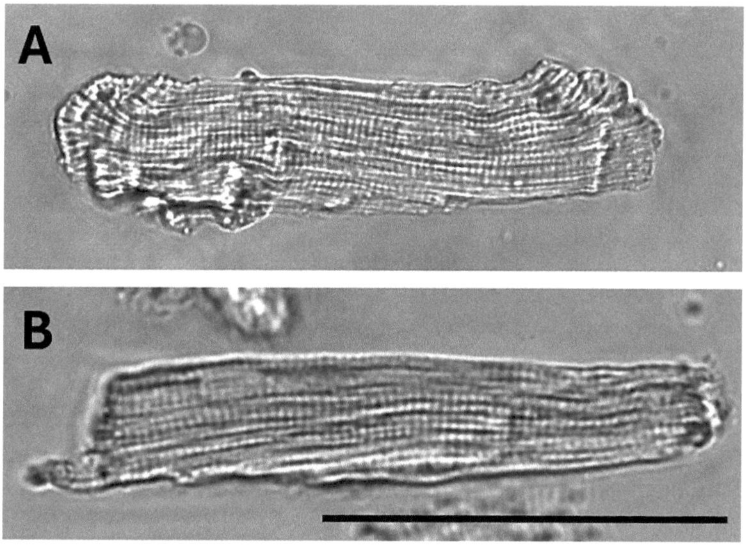

Fig. 3 Example of cells isolated using the described protocol. (**a**) Damaged cell, note rounded edges, blebs, and areas where striations are disturbed. This example cell also displayed spontaneous contractions. (**b**) Healthy cell, note clear striations and well-defined edges. Scale bar = 100 μm

4 Notes

1. The Langendorff apparatus allows for retrograde perfusion of the aorta and subsequent antegrade perfusion of the branching coronary arteries. The pressure of the solution keeps the aortic valve closed, while a suture prevents solution from exiting the aorta. Pressure can be generated by either a pump-based system offering constant flow or a hydrostatic/gravity-based system providing constant pressure. In our experience, constant pressure provides the best result and is easiest to optimize based on changes in flow rate as the heart becomes more digested. The Langendorff system consists of two 75 mL reservoirs located 90 cm above a cannula (Fig. 1). The reservoirs are connected to the perfusion system via peroxide silicone tubing (ID: 2.8 mm), through to a three-way valve. The three-way valve enables rapid switching of perfusion solutions. The height provides a perfusion pressure that generates an optimal flow rate through the coronary system for digestion to take place. The reservoirs are heated to ~37 °C via water jackets supplied by a water bath circulator. The water bath is set to 40 °C to heat the perfusion solutions to the required temperature. Pure O_2 is supplied to each reservoir via bubblers. A bubble trap heat exchanger device sits superior to the cannula to further control the temperature and avoid bubbles entering the heart. A 20 gauge blunt tip cannula with a circumferential notch

approximately 1.5 mm from the end is attached to the end for mounting of the heart. The blunt tip of the cannula is made by removing grinding the tip of a 20 gauge needle flat. The notch is created approximately 1.5 mm from the tip by a blade. The notch allows the aorta to be secured to the cannula with a braided silk suture.

2. The solutions used in this experiment should be made fresh on the day of the experiment. While some protocols filter all the solutions before use, we have not found this to be necessary. However, the use of MilliQ H_2O direct from the still is preferable compared to H_2O stored in containers for longer periods of time. We use a HEPES-buffered solution; therefore, the solution is gassed with O_2 rather than carbogen.
3. At any one time, Worthington Biochemical Corporation provides several batches/lots of collagenase type II with different enzymatic profiles. Depending on availability, users will likely need to trial more than one batch to determine the optimal enzymatic profile. Once a preference is determined, it is advisable to purchase a large volume of the lot to permit routine use without re-optimizing. Typically, batches containing higher protease activity, due a relatively higher level of clostripain (sulfhydryl protease), are preferable. The presence of a trypsin-like enzyme called aminopeptidase is also beneficial. The table below provides the characteristics of a batch that provided a large yield of cells and should form the basis for identifying suitable batches.
4. Ensure to check the reservoirs always have enough solution to prevent air entering the tubing.
5. Dropping the cannula low to the petri dish allows for a more successful transfer and prevents dropping of the heart. This method will also reduce the time the heart is out of solution. The apparatus can be lifted once the heart is secured.
6. Some protocols use heparin to reduce the formation of clots [15]; however, in our experience, this is not necessary if the cannulation and perfusion is completed quicky. Take note of the drip rate at this point; this will vary between experiments but should be approximately one drop every 3 s.
7. *See* Fig. 4.
8. Using a 3 mL transfer pipette with the tip cut off creates a wider bore that can be used for tissue trituration while the chunks are still relatively large.
9. If the tissue does not dissociate, this is a sign of under-digestion. Opposingly, if the tissue dissociates with no/little trituration, this is a sign of over-digestion. In these cases, the yield of viable cells is likely to be low, and the digestion time

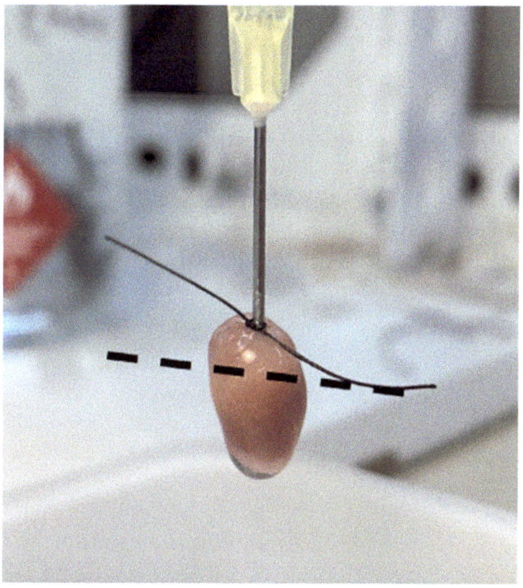

Fig. 4 Mouse heart attached to the cannula. Dashed line shows approximate place to cut the heart to collect the ventricles

during perfusion should be adjusted accordingly (increase time if under-digested, decrease time if over-digested).

10. Cardiomyocytes of a spherical shape are nonviable cells that have had their sarcolemma damaged due to "aggressive digestion" [16]. These cells will not display contractile activity. Other damaged cells will show spontaneous contractions.

References

1. Powell T, Twist V (1976) A rapid technique for the isolation and purification of adult cardiac muscle cells having respiratory control and a tolerance to calcium. Biochem Biophys Res Commun 72:327–333
2. Zhang H, Rabinovich PS (2022) Protocol for isolation of Cardiomyocyte from adult mouse and rat. Bio-prot 12:e4412–e4412
3. Feng J et al (2022) Methods of mouse cardiomyocyte isolation from postnatal heart. J Mol Cell Cardiol 168:35–43
4. Leone M, Engel FB (2021) Isolation, culture, and live-cell imaging of primary rat cardiomyocytes. Cardiac Regeneration Methods Protocol 1:109–124
5. Ackers-Johnson M et al (2016) A simplified, Langendorff-free method for concomitant isolation of viable cardiac myocytes and nonmyocytes from the adult mouse heart. Circ Res 199:909–920
6. Dobrev D et al (2000) G-protein β3-subunit 825T allele is associated with enhanced human atrial inward rectifier potassium currents. Circulation 102:692–697
7. Carneiro-Júnior MA et al (2013) The benefits of endurance training in cardiomyocyte function in hypertensive rats are reversed within four weeks of detraining. J Mol Cell Cardiol 57:119–128
8. Iribe G et al (2014) Load dependency in force-length relations in isolated single cardiomyocytes. Prog Biophys Mol Biol 115(2–3): 103–114
9. Gorski PA et al (2018) Measuring cardiomyocyte contractility and calcium handling in vitro. Exp Models Cardiovasc Dis Methods Protocol 1816:93 104
10. Waldeyer C et al (2009) Regional, age-dependent, and genotype-dependent differences in ventricular action potential duration and activation time in 410 Langendorff-perfused mouse hearts. Basic Res Cardiol 104: 523–533

11. Jackson SJ et al (2017) Does age matter? The impact of rodent age on study outcomes. Lab Anim 51:160–169
12. Feridooni HA et al (2017) The impact of age and frailty on ventricular structure and function in C57BL/6J mice. J Physiol 595:3721–3742
13. Zimmerman AN et al (1967) Morphological changes of heart muscle caused by successive perfusion with calcium-free and calcium-containing solutions (calcium paradox). Cardiovasc Res 1:201–209
14. Kao RL et al (1980) The effects of insulin and anoxia on the metabolism of isolated mature rat cardiac myocytes. Arch Biochem Biophys 203:587–599
15. O'Connell TD et al (2007) Isolation and culture of adult mouse cardiac myocytes. Cardiovasc Proteomics Methods Protocol 357:271–296
16. Thum T, Borlak J (2000) Isolation and cultivation of Ca2+ tolerant cardiomyocytes from the adult rat: improvements and applications. Xenobiotica 30:1063–1077

Chapter 3

Isolation of Endothelial Cells from Human Internal Mammary Artery

Puja Paudel, Fiona McDonald, and Martin Fronius

Abstract

Endothelial cells are a major contributor to cardiovascular diseases. Studying their function and how they influence pathological processes remains an ongoing area of research. Although primary endothelial cells might be readily available from animals, translating results from these studies can be challenging due to species-dependent differences. A common source of human endothelial cells is human umbilical vein endothelial cells, but these cells might not represent the variety of endothelial cells from various vascular beds. Here we describe a protocol for the isolation and cultivation of endothelial cells from human internal mammary artery remains. These remains are commonly available from coronary artery bypass graft surgeries. The described tissue explant method combined with a magnetic sorting process provided a relatively high yield of endothelial cells that were subsequently passaged and used for studies involving mRNA and protein expression analyses, as well as fluorescence-based immunohistochemistry and patch-clamp electrophysiology. This protocol may help to extend the repertoire of studying human endothelial cells to understand their role and function in health and disease.

Key words Endothelial cells, Primary cells, Internal mammary artery, Human tissue, Epithelial Na^+ channel, Vascular function

1 Introduction

Dysfunction of endothelial cells is one of the early hallmarks of cardiovascular diseases such as atherosclerosis, hypertension, and diabetes [1, 2]. Thus, research on endothelial cells provides information about risk factors associated with cardiovascular pathogenesis, and primary endothelial cells are important research tools as they closely mimic the in vivo conditions. Human umbilical cord vein endothelial cells (HUVECs) are one of the most widely used primary cell models for cardiovascular research due to their availability and accessibility [3, 4]. However, it is important to note that there is marked phenotypic variation between endothelial cells from various vascular origins [5]. Due to the origin from the umbilical cord vein, HUVECs might not be the ideal cell model to mimic the

Dhananjie N. K. Chandrasekera and Rajesh Katare (eds.), *Cardiomyocytes: Methods and Protocols*, Methods in Molecular Biology, vol. 2894, https://doi.org/10.1007/978-1-0716-4342-6_3,

in vivo physiology of adult vasculature. Alternatively, primary endothelial cells isolated from animal arteries can be used. However, in some cases, species-dependent differences limit the translation of the findings into clinical settings. An example for this is represented by the expression and function of epithelial sodium channel (ENaC) proteins in the vasculature and endothelial cells. Besides its role for maintaining Na^+ and water homeostasis via its function in the kidneys [6], ENaC is expressed in endothelial cells [7] and is involved in blood pressure regulation by mediating vascular responsiveness [8]. There are four ENaC genes in humans (*SCNN1A*, *SCNN1B*, *SCNN1G*, *SCNN1D*), encoding four ENaC protein subunits (α, β, γ, and δ). These proteins commonly assemble as trimers in combinations of αβγ- or δβγ-ENaC to form functional channels (reviewed in [9]). The gene encoding the δ-ENaC subunit is a pseudogene in rats and mice which are commonly used in preclinical biomedical research [10, 11]. Thus, the δ-ENaC protein is not expressed in these common animal models. The detection of the δ-ENaC subunit in HUVECs [12] highlights the necessity for human endothelial cells to further this area of research. However, the availability of human arteries for the isolation of endothelial cells is a limitation. Therefore, we have explored the use of human internal mammary arteries (IMA) for isolating and cultivating primary endothelial cells. These arteries are commonly used for coronary artery bypass graft surgery (CABG), and the remaining tissues not needed for surgery are readily accessible.

There are two common approaches to obtain endothelial cells from fresh arteries: (1) enzymatic tissue digestion [13] and (2) tissue explant [14]. In our case, enzymatic digestion did not yield sufficient endothelial cells for successful culture and subsequent analyses and the purity of cells was poor. However, the tissue explant method combined with gelatin-coated dishes provided high yields and a purer population of endothelial cells which was successfully used to characterize ENaC subunit expression at gene and protein level and ENaC function by patch-clamp electrophysiology in human endothelial cells originating from IMA [15]. The method is also applicable for small segments of arteries (e.g., aortic punches), but it should be considered that the total amount of cells obtained correlates with the size of tissue available from the surgery. Although the protocol presented here has been specifically developed to study the role of ENaC in human endothelial cells, it offers a translational perspective for vascular research using human cells that are easily available and represent a step toward personalized medicine.

Postsurgically discarded segments of human IMA were used for the study. Patients provided written informed consent prior to surgery, and the use of human arterial tissues was approved by the Health and Disability Ethics Committee in New Zealand (LRS/12/01/001/AM17). The arterial segments not needed for the CABG procedure were collected in the operation theatre and transferred immediately to the laboratory where the procedures outlined below were performed (*see* **Note 1**).

2 Materials

The following materials were used for the isolation and verification of endothelial cells isolated from internal mammary arteries. All solutions must be prepared under sterile conditions and equipment such as scissors and forceps should be autoclaved before use.

2.1 Tissue Collection and Dissection (See Notes 2 and 7)

1. Ice-cold Hank's Balanced Salt Solution (HBSS, Sigma-Aldrich): 0.35 g/L $NaHCO_3$, 1.0 g/L glucose.
2. Heparin sodium salt (1000 U/mL, Sigma-Aldrich).
3. 1% penicillin/streptomycin (Gibco).
4. Autoclaved fine forceps.
5. Autoclaved scissors.
6. 100 mm petri dish.

2.2 Tissue Explant Reagents (See Note 3)

1. 35 mm petri dishes.
2. Phosphate buffer solution (PBS, Gibco): 155 mM NaCl, 2.7 mM Na_2HPO_4, and 1.5 mM KH_2PO_4.
3. 1% gelatin (Sigma-Aldrich).
4. Endothelial growth medium (EGM-2, Lonza). Specific medium was used because it includes nutrients, growth factors, and hormones tailored for endothelial cells.
5. EGM-2 bulletkit (Lonza): 25 mL fetal bovine serum (FBS), 0.2 mL hydrocortisone, 2 mL hFGF-B, 0.5 mL VEGF, 0.5 mL R3-IGF-1, 0.5 mL ascorbic acid, 0.5 mL hEGF, 0.5 mL GA-1000.
6. Fetal bovine serum (FBS, Gibco).
7. 1% penicillin/streptomycin.

2.3 Endothelial Cell Sorting (See Note 4)

1. PBS (Sigma-Aldrich): 155 mM NaCl, 2.7 mM Na_2HPO_4, and 1.5 mM KH_2PO_4.
2. Trypsin–EDTA (Gibco).
3. Dulbecco's Phosphate Buffered Saline (DPBS, Sigma-Aldrich): 138 mM NaCl 2.7 mM KCl, 1.5 mM KH_2PO_4, 8 mM Na_2HPO_4.
4. Bovine serum albumin (BSA, Thermo Fisher).
5. Anti-CD31 microbeads (Miltenyi Biotech).
6. FcR blocking reagent (Miltenyi Biotech).

7. MACS Multistand (Miltenyi Biotech).
8. MidiMACS Separator (Miltenyi Biotech).
9. LS columns (Miltenyi Biotech).

2.4 Cell Culture After Cell Sorting

1. EGM-2 basal medium.
2. EGM-2 bulletkit.
3. 10% FBS.
4. 1% penicillin/streptomycin.

2.5 Reagents for Immunofluorescence (See Note 5)

1. PBS: 155 mM NaCl, 2.7 mM Na_2HPO_4, and 1.5 mM KH_2PO_4.
2. 4% formaldehyde (Sigma-Aldrich) in PBS.
3. 0.25% Triton X-100 (Sigma-Aldrich).
4. Blocking buffer: 4% (w/v) BSA and 5% (w/v) normal goat serum in 50 mL PBS (137 mM NaCl, 2.7 mM KCl, 10 mM Na_2HPO_4, and 1.8 mM KH_2PO_4).
5. Anti-CD31 antibody (Invitrogen, dilution 1:100).
6. Alexafluor-488 (Abcam, 1:200).
7. VECTASHIELD® Hard Set Mounting medium with DAPI (Vector Laboratories).
8. 12 mm coverslips.
9. 0.2% gelatin (Marienfeld).
10. 24-well plates.
11. Fluorescence microscope for imaging.

2.6 Reagents for Tube Formation Assay

1. Matrigel® matrix (Corning).
2. 96-well plate.
3. Pre-cooled pipette tips.
4. Light microscope for imaging.

3 Methods

3.1 Tissue Collection, Dissection, and Explant

1. Arterial tissue not further needed for the graft to be placed in a tube containing 5 mL of ice-cold HBBS on ice and transferred from the operating room to the laboratory to start the isolation process (Fig. 1, *see* **Note 1**). Start the isolation process as soon as possible but not longer than 2 h after transfer from the operating theatre, to retain viability of the tissue and cells.
2. Warm a tube of complete EGM-2 media to 37 °C in the water bath.

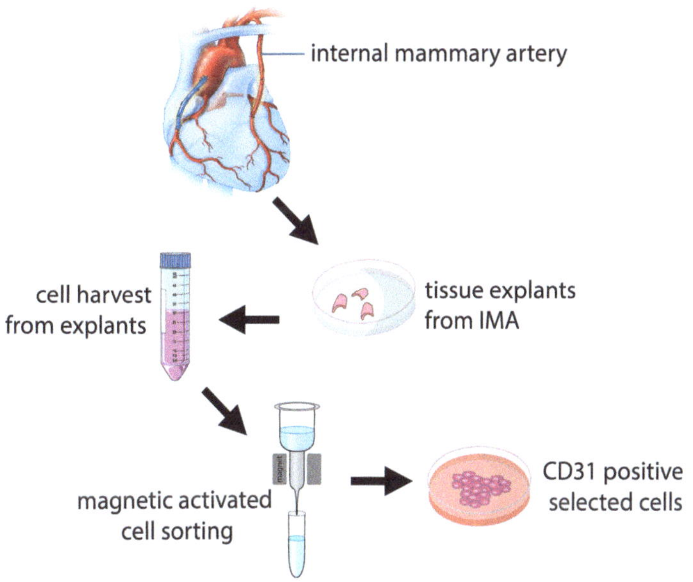

Fig. 1 Overview of the protocol for the isolation and purification of primary endothelial cells from human internal mammary artery remains available from coronary artery bypass graft surgeries. Human arteries are cut into small pieces and incubated with endothelial side downward on gelatin-coated plates. The endothelial cells divide and migrate out from the tissue explant and can be harvested from the plates. Cell suspensions can then be subjected to a cell sorting process to obtain endothelial cells

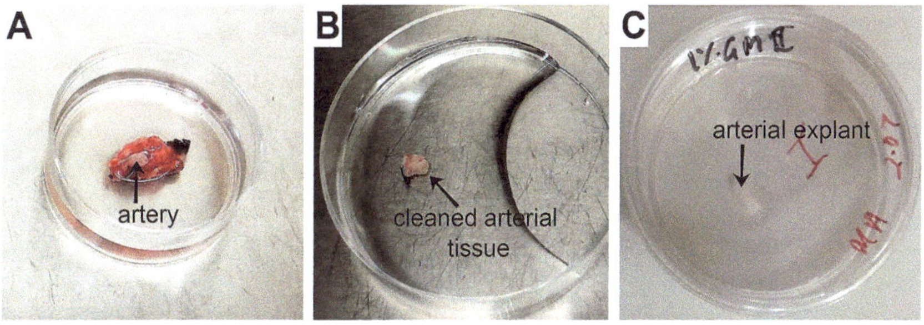

Fig. 2 Preparation of IMA remains for arterial explants. (**a**) The arterial tissue with attached muscles and adipose tissues from the hospital. (**b**) Arterial tissue after the removal of excess muscle and adipose tissues. (**c**) A cleaned arterial explant placed lumen side down onto a gelatin-coated dish

3. Transfer the arterial tissue segment to a 100 mm petri dish filled with fresh ice-cold HBBS buffer (Fig. 2a).
4. Wash the arterial segment with ice-cold HBBS three times.
5. Using the autoclaved scissors and forceps, remove muscle and adipose tissues and wash again two times with the ice-cold HBSS to remove blood or remaining tissue pieces (Fig. 2b).

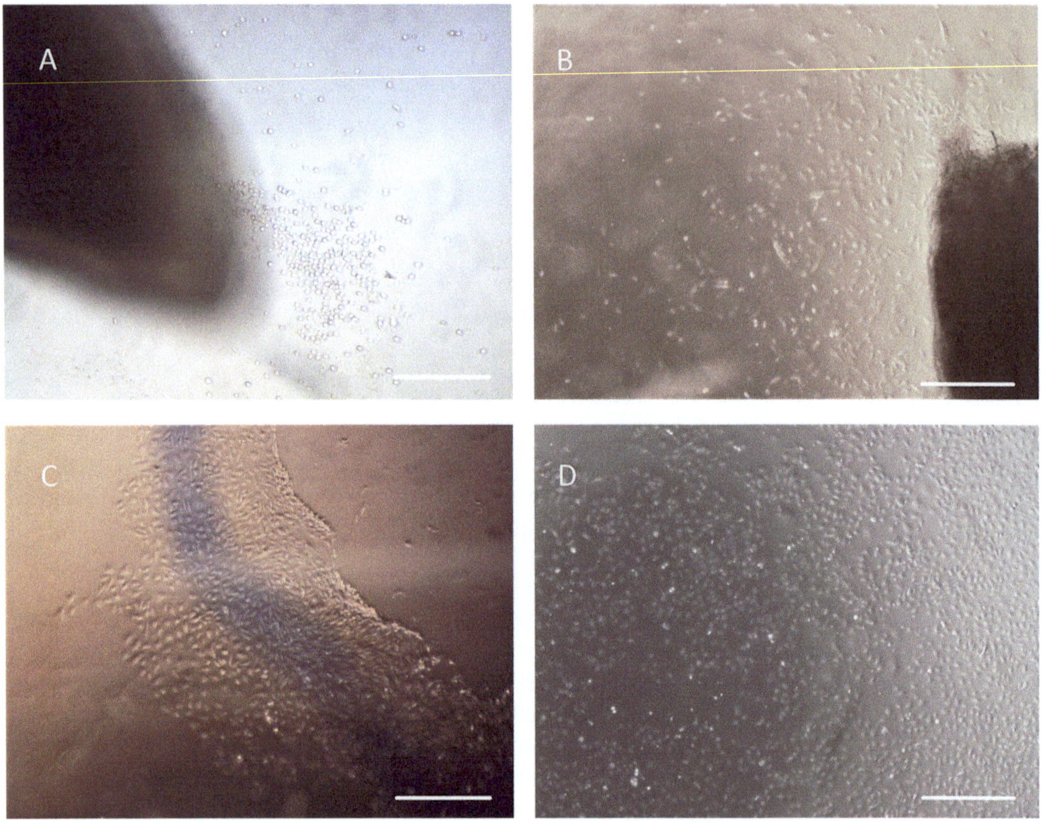

Fig. 3 Series of microscopy images of arterial explants and cell outgrowth from IMA. (**a**) IMA explant on day two. (**b**) Cell outgrowth and migration from the arterial explant on day seven. (**c**) Vascular cells after removal of the arterial explant on day ten. (**d**) Semi-confluent cells cultured on day fourteen. Scale bar = 0.5 mm

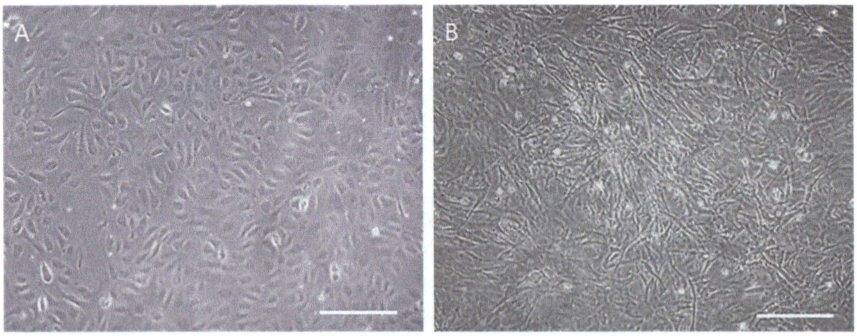

Fig. 4 Primary cells from IMA after cell sorting with MACS magnetic microbeads. (**a**) Cells obtained following magnetic cell sorting representing the CD31 positive fraction. (**b**) Cells obtained from the same process but representing the fraction of cells passing through the column (CD31 negative). These cells have a elongated spindle-shape morphology and are likely fibroblasts. CD31 positive and -negative cells are easily distinguished by their appearance. Scale bar = 0.2 mm

6. Place the artery segment in a new 100 mm petri dish filled with fresh HBSS and cut the artery open to expose the inner endothelial layer.
7. Dissect the arterial tissue into 2–3 mm segments. The number of obtained segments may depend on the size of arterial tissue provided.
8. Using fine forceps, transfer the artery segment into a 35 mm petri dish with the luminal side facing downward toward the gelatin-coated bottom of the dish (Fig. 2c). Use two to three segments per petri dish.
9. Place each plate covered with a lid into an incubator (37 °C for 5 min) to let the tissue attach to the plate. This prevents the detachment of artery segments when media is added. The incubation should not be too long to prevent desiccation of the tissue segments.
10. Remove the petri dishes from the incubator and gently add 500 μL of the warmed complete EGM-2 media (20% FBS) to each dish (*see* **Note 3** for media preparation). The media should cover the tissue segments but their detachment from the bottom of the dish should be avoided (*see* **Note 6**).
11. With the lids on, carefully transfer the petri dishes to an incubator (37 °C and 5% CO_2) and leave for 24 h.
12. Change the media after 24 h to remove dead cells. Arterial segments should be kept wet all the time and detachment from the bottom of the plate should be avoided. The explants should be monitored with a microscope (Fig. 3) to observe the outgrowth of cells from the explant and placed back into the incubator. Subsequently, every 24 h, the media should be changed, and explants should be checked for contamination (*see* **Note 7**).
13. After ~7 days, cells start to migrate out of the explant. Once cells migrating out of arterial explant can be observed (Fig. 3), the medium should be changed to the complete medium containing 10% FBS (instead of 20% FBS).
14. On day 9, use autoclaved fine forceps to gently remove and discard the tissue segment. Cells should remain attached to the petri dish bottom. Add 1.5 mL of complete EGM-2 media (10% FBS) and transfer the petri dish back to the incubator. Repeat this daily and monitor if fibroblasts can be observed (elongated, spindle-shaped cells) and distinguished from endothelial cells (Fig. 4). If fibroblast contamination is excessive, discard the dish.

3.2 Endothelial Cell Isolation and Sorting

1. Approximately 15–18 days after surgery, the endothelial cells should have grown to ~50–60% confluency and can be isolated for a sorting process. Therefore, PBS, trypsin–EDTA, and complete EGM-2 should be warmed to 37 °C.
2. Transfer the dishes containing the cells to the biosafety cabinet and aspirate the media. Rinse the cells twice with PBS to remove the residual medium and cell debris.
3. Add 1 mL warm trypsin–EDTA to each dish and incubate the cells for 5 min at 37 °C to detach the cells from the dish bottom. Then check under a microscope if cells have detached from the dish and if not, gently tap against the side of the plate to detach the cells.
4. Once cells are suspended, add 3 mL complete EGM-2 media to neutralize the action of trypsin–EDTA and transfer the cells to a 15 mL tube. Spin the tube in a centrifuge at 500 rpm for 5 min to collect the cells at the bottom of the tube.
5. Carefully aspirate the supernatant to obtain a cell pellet. The cells can now be frozen and stored for future use or passaged to increase cell numbers and subjected to magnetic cell sorting to obtain a high purity of endothelial cells.

3.3 Cell Passaging

1. Resuspend the cell pellet by adding 1 mL complete medium.
2. Gently pipette up and down ~3–4 times.
3. Transfer the cell suspension to a gelatin-coated cell culture flask and incubate as described before (**step 14** of Subheading 3.1).

3.4 Magnetic Activated Cell Sorting

1. Resuspend the cell pellet with 1 mL of fresh, ice-cold DPBS wash buffer. Centrifuge the cells at 500 rpm for 5 min and carefully aspirate the supernatant.
2. Resuspend the cells to a maximum concentration of 1×10^7 cells per 60 μL DPBS washing buffer as advised by the manufacturer's protocol (Miltenyi Biotech). Add 20 μL of FcR blocking reagent per 1×10^7 cells. Mix well by pipetting up and down a few times. Add 20 μL of CD31 microbeads to the cell suspension and mix well by further pipetting.
3. Incubate the cells for 15 min at 4 °C.
4. Add 1 mL of DPBS wash buffer before centrifuging at 500 rpm for 3 min.
5. Discard the supernatant and resuspend the cell pellet in 2 mL of DPBS wash buffer.
6. Place the LS column in the magnetic field and rinse it with 3 mL of DPBS wash buffer. Discard the buffer.

7. Transfer the cell suspension onto the column. Collect the flow-through cells. These cells are expected to be CD31 negative and are considered as non-endothelial cells.
8. Wash the column five times with 1 mL of DPBS wash buffer for each time to remove unlabeled cells from the column.
9. Remove the column from the separator and magnet and place it on a collection tube.
10. Add 1 mL of DPBS wash buffer onto the column to flush out the magnetically labeled cells from the column. Do this by firmly pushing the plunger into the column. The obtained cells are CD31-positive cells and are expected to represent endothelial cells. With immunofluorescence detection for CD31 (see steps below), we were able to obtain a cell population that was ~90% CD31 positive.
11. Centrifuge the collector tube at 4 °C and 500 rpm for 8 min and aspirate the supernatant completely. Finally, resuspend the cells in complete EGM-2 media (*see* **step 1** of Subheading 3.3).
12. Transfer the cells to a 0.2% gelatin-coated petri dish and incubate at the abovementioned culture condition.

3.5 Characterization of Cells by Immunofluorescence

1. Place 12 mm coverslips coated with gelatin into a 24-well plate and seed 1 × 10^4 cells per coverslip in 400 μL of complete EGM-2 media and incubate at 37 °C in a humidified atmosphere of 5% CO_2.
2. After 24 h of incubation, rinse the cells three times with warm PBS and fix the cells by adding PBS containing 4% formaldehyde for 20 min at room temperature.
3. Remove formaldehyde and rinse the cells three times with ice-cold PBS. Then permeabilize the cells by adding 0.25% Triton X-100 diluted in PBS for 10 min at room temperature.
4. Rinse the cells three times with ice-cold PBS (300 μL per well/slide). Leave the PBS for each rinse for 5 min before aspirating. During this time, prepare the blocking solution and a humidified chamber that is lined with a wet paper towel.
5. After the last washing step, aspirate the PBS and carefully transfer the coverslips onto the top of a microscopic slide. Cover the slides with blocking buffer and incubate for 1 h at room temperature within the humidified chamber.
6. Take the microscope slides from the chamber and carefully remove the blocking buffer from the coverslips using a pipette.
7. Treat the cells with primary antibody diluted in blocking buffer and incubate the slides at 4 °C overnight.
8. Rinse the cells three times for 5 min each with ice-cold PBS and then incubate the cells with the secondary antibody for 1 h at room temperature.

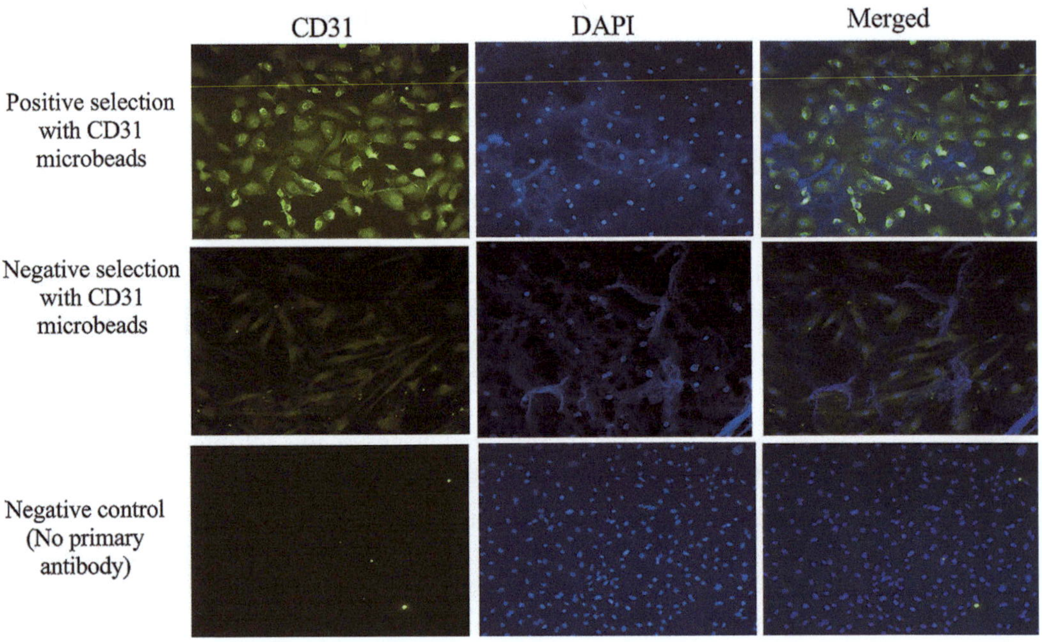

Fig. 5 Fluorescent microscopy images from CD31 positive and -negative cells following magnetic sorting. Expression of CD31 was detected using anti-CD31 antibody and Alexafluor-488 conjugated antibody (green). The nuclei were stained with DAPI (blue, n = 4, Scale bar: 0.2 mm)

9. Rinse the cells three times for 5 min each with PBS. Dispense VECTASHIELD® on top of the coverslip and leave at room temperature for 15 min. Finalize the process by incubating the coverslips overnight at 4 °C in the dark. The following day, the images can be taken under a fluorescence microscope (Fig. 5).

3.6 Tube Formation Assay

In addition to the detection of CD31, a tube formation assay can be performed to assess the angiogenic properties of the isolated cells (Fig. 6).

1. Thaw Matrigel matrix (Corning) on ice and place a 96-well plate on ice (*see* **Note 8**). Once the Matrigel has liquified, add 100 μL of Matrigel per well used. Use a pre-cooled pipette tip to avoid solidifying the Matrigel (which occurs at room temperature) and swirl the plate to distribute the Matrigel evenly.
2. Incubate the plate at 37 °C for at least 30 min and remove excess solution if present, without disturbing the solidified coat. The plate is now ready to use.
3. Resuspend the trypsinized cells (as described before) and count the cells. Add 1×10^4 cells per well of the Matrigel-coated plate and transfer the cells to the incubator at 37 °C and 5% CO_2 atmosphere.

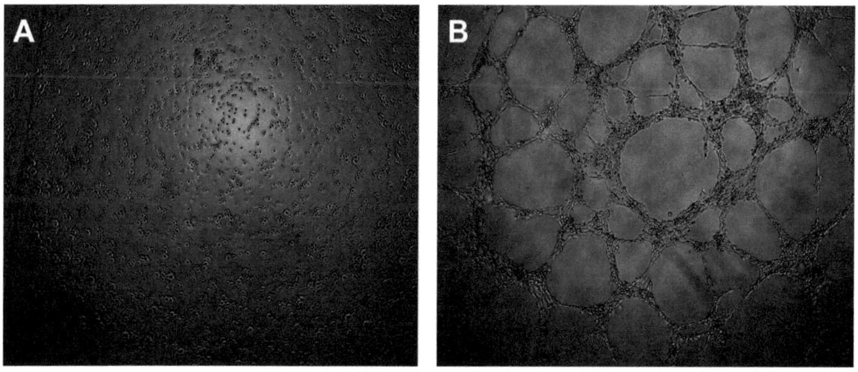

Fig. 6 Representative image of in-vitro tube formation assay of cells isolated from IMA. Images were taken at (**a**) 0 hours and (**b**) 8 hours of the assay. Cells used for the depicted assay were from passage 5 and were cultured in a matrigel matrix. The tube formation suggests that the cells retained their endothelial phenotype even after passaging (n = 4)

4. Examine the plate under a microscope and take images of the cells at 0, 2, 4, 8, and 16 h (or as desired). The formation of tubelike structures was observed as early as 2 h after plating the cells on Matrigel and appeared to be completed after ~8 h.

4 Notes

1. Timely processing of the extracted tissue has been observed to be beneficial for a good yield of cells. Key elements for this are adequate preparation of required reagents in advance and reassuring that access to cell culture hoods and other resources is in place. Further, good and dependable communication with the surgical team is essential. This also ensures timely transfer of tissues from the surgical theatre and quick processing of the tissues to maximize yield of cell harvest.
2. Ice-cold Hank's Balanced Salt Solution (HBSS) should be supplemented with heparin sodium salt (1000 U/mL), and 1% penicillin/streptomycin should be stored on ice for the collection of the tissue. Autoclaved fine forceps and scissors (FST) are required for the removal of adipose and muscle tissues. A dissection microscope can be helpful for this process. After removal of connective tissues, the artery can be cut open to form a flat sheet. These are then dissected into small segments (2–3 mm).
3. 35 mm petri dishes (Greiner) should be coated with PBS (phosphate-buffered solution, Sigma-Aldrich) supplemented with 1% gelatin (Sigma-Aldrich). The endothelial cell-specific medium for the extraction for cultivating the explant segments should be prepared in advance and aliquoted for future use.

Therefore, the endothelial growth medium (EGM-2, Lonza) should be supplemented with EGM-2 bulletkit (Lonza) as per the manufacturer's instructions, including 10% FBS and 1% penicillin/streptomycin. Aliquots containing 50 mL in Falcon tubes should be prepared that can be stored at 4 °C for future use. One aliquot should be prepared with 20% FBS, that will be used initially, until cell migration is observed (~day 7). After this, medium aliquots with 10% FBS are used. Media must always be pre-warmed to 37 °C before use.

4. Warmed PBS, 0.25% trypsin–EDTA combined with cultivating medium to neutralize the trypsin should be used for cell isolation from the explants. For cell sorting, Dulbecco's Phosphate-Buffered Saline (DPBS) supplemented with 0.5% (w/v) BSA (bovine serum albumin) was used as washing buffer for this protocol. This washing buffer should be prepared fresh for each cell sorting procedure. Cell sorting was achieved using magnetic activated cell sorting (MACS®) reagents and materials sourced from Miltenyi Biotec including anti-CD31 microbeads, FcR blocking reagent, MACS Multistand, MidiMACS Separator, and LS columns.
5. VECTASHIELD® Hard Set Mounting medium with DAPI (Vector Laboratories) was used to preserve the samples for immunofluorescence. Cells were grown on 12 mm coverslips coated with 0.2% gelatin (Marienfeld) placed in 24-well plates.
6. To avoid detachment of tissues, the media should be added slowly and carefully. The pipette tip might be directed toward the verge of the petri dish, not toward the tissues. Gently tilt the petri dish to distribute the solution evenly within the dish.
7. Particular care needs to be taken to avoid contamination during the transfer processes from the operating theatre to the cell culture facility and the processing of the tissue for cultivation. All solutions (e.g., PBS), used in the process, should be passed through a 0.2 μm sterile filter membrane. Other instruments and dishes need to be autoclaved before use.
8. Thaw Matrigel matrix one day before use at 4 °C. Pre-cool 96-well plate and pipette tips overnight in the refrigerator. Added 25 μL of Matrigel matrix to the required number of wells of the precooled 96-well culture plate. Place the 96-well plate containing the Matrigel matrix for 30 min in an incubator at 37 °C to solidify. During this time, the cultured primary endothelial cells should be trypsinized and centrifuged.

Acknowledgements

This work was supported by a PhD scholarship from the Department of Physiology, University of Otago, Dunedin, New Zealand. We want to express our gratitude to the patients, who provided consent to allow the collection of arterial tissues that was used for the study. Further, we are thankful for the support of the surgical team at Dunedin Hospital that enabled the collection of the tissues and Isabell van Hout, who was crucial for overseeing the cooperation between the surgical team and the scientists and for coordinating the transfers of tissues to the research lab.

Author Contribution P.P. developed the protocol, performed the experiments, analyzed the data, and wrote the manuscript. M.F. and F.J.M. supervised the project and provided feedback throughout the writing of the manuscript. P.P. and M.F. finalized and submitted the manuscript.

References

1. Knapp M, Tu X, Wu R (2019) Vascular endothelial dysfunction, a major mediator in diabetic cardiomyopathy. Acta Pharmacol Sin 40:1–8
2. Taddei S, Virdis A, Ghiadoni L, Sudano I, Salvetti A (2001) Endothelial dysfunction in hypertension. J Cardiovasc Pharmacol 38 (Suppl 2):S11–S14
3. Marin V, Kaplanski G, Grès S, Farnarier C, Bongrand P (2001) Endothelial cell culture: protocol to obtain and cultivate human umbilical endothelial cells. J Immunol Methods 254:183–190
4. Park HJ, Zhang Y, Georgescu SP, Johnson KL, Kong D, Galper JB (2006) Human umbilical vein endothelial cells and human dermal microvascular endothelial cells offer new insights into the relationship between lipid metabolism and angiogenesis. Stem Cell Rev 2:93–102
5. Aird WC (2007) Phenotypic heterogeneity of the endothelium: I. Structure, function, and mechanisms. Circ Res 100:158–173
6. Garty H, Palmer LG (1997) Epithelial sodium channels: function, structure, and regulation. Physiol Rev 77:359–396
7. Kusche-Vihrog K, Callies C, Fels J, Oberleithner H (2010) The epithelial sodium channel (ENaC): mediator of the aldosterone response in the vascular endothelium. Steroids 75:544–549
8. Ashley Z, Mugloo S, McDonald FJ, Fronius M (2018) Epithelial Na+ channel differentially contributes to shear stress-mediated vascular responsiveness in carotid and mesenteric arteries from mice. Am J Physiol Heart Circ Physiol 314:H1022–H1032
9. Hanukoglu I, Hanukoglu A (2016) Epithelial sodium channel (ENaC) family: phylogeny, structure-function, tissue distribution, and associated inherited diseases. Gene 579:95–132
10. Gettings SM, Maxeiner S, Tzika M, Cobain MRD, Ruf I, Benseler F, Brose N, Krasteva-Christ G, Vande Velde G, Schönberger M, Althaus M (2021) Two functional epithelial sodium channel isoforms are present in rodents despite pronounced evolutionary pseudogenisation and exon fusion. Mol Biol Evol 38: msab271
11. Giraldez T, Rojas P, Jou J, Flores C, Alvarez de la Rosa D (2012) The epithelial sodium channel delta-subunit: new notes for an old song. Am J Physiol Renal Physiol 303:F328–F338
12. Downs CA, Johnson NM, Coca C, Helms MN (2017) Angiotensin II regulates δ-ENaC in

human umbilical vein endothelial cells. Microvasc Res 116:26–33
13. Wang J, Niu N, Xu S, Jin ZG (2019) A simple protocol for isolating mouse lung endothelial cells. Sci Rep 9:1458
14. Choi S, Kim JA, Kim KC, Suh SH (2015) Isolation and in vitro culture of vascular endothelial cells from mice. Korean J Physiol Pharmacol 19:35–42
15. Paudel P, van Hout I, Bunton RW, Parry DJ, Coffey S, McDonald FJ, Fronius M (2022) Epithelial Sodium Channel δ subunit is expressed in human arteries and has potential association with hypertension. Hypertension 79:1385–1394

Chapter 4

Mitochondrial Membrane Potential and Lactate Dehydrogenase Activity in a Model of Acute In Vitro Ischemia/Reperfusion Injury

Deepthi Ashok, Haley Garbus, and Obialunanma V. Ebenebe

Abstract

Experimental models of cardiac ischemia/reperfusion injury have served as useful tools in isolating the sequence of events and mechanisms involved following an infarct. The in vitro coverslip ischemia model in neonatal myocytes is key in observing acute cellular and organelle changes during ischemia and in reperfusion. Here we use neonatal mouse ventricular myocytes, and describe two experimental readouts of lactate dehydrogenase assay, for cell damage/injury and measurement of mitochondrial membrane potential.

Key words Acute ischemia/reperfusion, Neonatal mouse ventricular myocytes, Cell culture, Mitochondria potential

1 Introduction

The compounding adverse effect of a myocardial infarction or myocardial ischemic event occurs following the removal of the initial infarct. This secondary phase of injury, caused by reperfusion of the infarcted area, has been an area of study for over 60 decades. First described in research in 1960 by Jennings et al. [1], the study of ischemia/reperfusion (I/R) injury has since aided the field of cardiovascular research by informing various sections of the underlying molecular changes which feed the overall pathology. Since Jennings' first report of this in dogs, there have been various experimental models devised to further isolate the chain of events following ischemia. These experimental models, usually in rodents and large mammals, range from in vivo ligation of the coronary artery [2, 3] to ex vivo global ischemia on the Langendorff system [4] to the most recently described of the three, in vitro coverslip

All authors are contributed equally to this work.

Dhananjie N. K. Chandrasekera and Rajesh Katare (eds.), *Cardiomyocytes: Methods and Protocols*, Methods in Molecular Biology, vol. 2894, https://doi.org/10.1007/978-1-0716-4342-6_4,

ischemia model [5]. Each of these methods has its advantages and disadvantages, and relevance will depend on the mechanistic aspect one is looking to investigate. This chapter will focus on the in vitro coverslip ischemia model initially developed by Pitts and Tombs in neonatal rat ventricular myocytes. The protocol described here utilizes neonatal mouse ventricular myocytes (NMVMs). Two experimental readouts will be described—a lactate dehydrogenase assay, which measures cell damage/injury to plasma membrane, and mitochondrial membrane potential using a cationic dye called tetramethylrhodamine methyl ester (TMRM) which sequesters into energetically coupled mitochondria. One advantage of this model is the ability to investigate the effect of various compounds on NMVM recovery post-ischemia (LDH assay) and any mitochondrial effects (via the TMRM fluorescence).

2 Materials

2.1 Fibronectin-Coated Plates

1. 15 mL conical tube.
2. Fibronectin bovine plasma: Weigh out 300 mg of fibronectin and dissolve according to manufacturer's instructions 10 mL of water (*see* **Note 3**). Filter-sterilize the solution and store in 4 °C until use.
3. Ultrapure sterile water.
4. 35 mm (D = 20 mm) glass coverslip dish.

2.2 Media

1. Isolation media: Medium 199 was supplemented with 25 mM HEPES, 2 ug/mL vitamin B12, 50 U/mL pen-strep, 1× non-essential 286 amino acids and 10% fetal bovine serum (FBS). Prepare vitamin B12 solution in dark (*see* **Note 1**): weigh out 10 mg of vitamin B12, dissolve in 10 mL of ultrapure sterile water, sterile filter, aliquot, and store at −20 °C in dark/amber tubes.
2. Cell culture media: Medium 199 was used as described above with 2% FBS instead.

2.3 Isolation

1. Magnetic activated cell sorting (MACS) separator with m_neo-heart_01 program (Miltenyi).
2. Magnetic stand.
3. Neonatal Heart Dissociation Kit—mouse, and rat: 2.3 mL Buffer X, 62.5 μL Enzyme P, 25 μL Buffer Y, 12.5 μL Enzyme A, and 100 μL Enzyme D, vortex-mix, and store at 8 °C until use.
4. Neonatal cardiomyocyte magnetic beads, mouse.
5. MS columns.

6. C-tube.
7. Water bath (37 °C).
8. 70 μm cell strainer.
9. Centrifuge.
10. MACS buffer: 100 mL 1× PBS, 0.5% bovine serum albumin (BSA), 2 mM EDTA.
11. Sterile dissection tools.
12. ACK lysis buffer: 15 mM ammonium chloride, 10 mM potassium bicarbonate, 0.1 mM EDTA.

2.4 Experimental Readouts

2.4.1 Lactate Dehydrogenase (LDH) Assay

1. CyQUANT LDH Cytotoxicity Assay.
2. Colorimetric plate reader: read at 490 nm and 680 nm absorbance.
3. 96-well plate.
4. Orbital shaker.
5. 1% bovine serum albumin in 1× PBS.
6. Multichannel pipette.

2.4.2 Mitochondrial Membrane Potential (MMP)

1. 10 μM tetramethylrhodamine methyl ester (TMRM) working stock solution made in sterile water.
2. Tyrode buffer: 130 mM NaCl, 5 mM KCl, 1 mM MgCl2, 10 mM NaHEPES, 1 mM $CaCl_2$, and 5 mM glucose.
3. Laser-scanning confocal microscope (Olympus FV3000RS).
4. 40× silicone-immersion objective (Olympus UPLSAPO40XS).

   Setting: 561 nm excitation/570–620 nm emission

   Galvano scanning mode.

   Laser intensity—0.06% power (20 mW 561 nm LED laser) (*see* **Note 2**).

   Images were 16 bits with a size of 318.2 × 319.2 microns (512 × 512 pixels).
5. Fiji ImageJ software: custom-built segmentation-analysis macro was generated to track each cell's MMP during the ischemia/reperfusion protocol.

   For analysis, the set of macros can be downloaded from https://github.com/dashok1/MitoWave/tree/v1.0.2.

3 Methods

All procedures should be completed underneath a sterile biosafety cabinet at room temperature unless otherwise specified. All solutions and equipment must be sterile. Use of appropriate aseptic technique is mandatory.

3.1 Preparation of Culture Plates

1. Add 1–2 mL of sterile fibronectin solution to bottom of glass plates ensuring the entire surface is covered.
2. Incubate prepared plates at 37 °C for a minimum of 2 h.

3.2 Dissection and Cell Isolation

1. Rinse five to six pups in 70% ethanol followed by sterile 1× PBS.
2. Euthanize pups by decapitation (*see* **Note 4**).
3. Once the heart has been dissected, rinse in ice-cold PBS (*see* **Note 5**).
4. Transfer heart into C-tube containing 2.5 mL of enzyme mix and mince (cut into three to four pieces).
5. Incubate in 37 °C water bath for 15 min without agitation.
6. Run column through MACS program: m_neoheart_01.
7. Repeat **steps 5** and **6** in sequence—total three times.
8. Add 15 mL of ice-cold *isolation media* (Subheading 2.2).
9. Strain through 70 μm cell strainer, and wash with 2–3 mL of *isolation media* (Subheading 2.2).
10. Centrifuge at 600 g for 5 min at 4 °C and discard the supernatant.
11. Resuspend pellet with 400 μL ACK lysis buffer and incubate for 5 min.
12. Add 10 mL of ice-cold MACS buffer (*see* **Note 6**).
13. Centrifuge at 300 g for 5 min at 4 °C and discard the supernatant.
14. Resuspend pellet in 1 mL MACS buffer and count cells.
15. Centrifuge at 300 g for 5 min at 4 °C.
16. Resuspend cells in appropriate volume of MACS buffer for 5×10^6 NMVMs in 90 μL.

3.2.1 Preparation of Column and Samples

1. Add 10 μL magnetic beads (130–100-825) to 90 uL of 5×10^6 NMVMs.
2. Incubate for 15 min at 4 °C.
3. Place MS column in MACS separator.
4. Pre-rinse MS column with 500 μL MACS buffer.

3.2.2 Cell Separation

1. Following NMVMs and bead mix incubation, add more volume of MACS buffer for a total volume of 500 μL.
2. Apply 500 μL of NMVMs and bead mix to MS column and collect flow-through in newly labeled tubes (*see* **Note 7**).
3. Repeat the above step as necessary depending on the sample number with a fresh MS column every 12–15 pups.

4. Rinse column after last samples with MACS buffer—to collect residual NMVMs.
5. Count newly collected NMVMs.
6. Centrifuge and resuspend in 400 μL of *isolation media* for 1×10^6 cells.

3.2.3 Plating Cells

1. Wash fibronectin-coated glass coverslip dishes with pre-warmed *isolation media* once.
2. Plate 400 μL of 1×10^6cells onto dish.
3. Store in a sterile incubator at usual conditions (95% O_2, 5% CO_2, 37 °C) overnight.
4. Next day, change media to 2 mL of *cell culture media* (containing 2% FBS; *2.2*) and maintain NMVMs until ischemia/reperfusion (I/R) experiments.
5. I/R experiments and imaging are performed between 4 and 6 days of isolation.

3.3 Ischemia/ Reperfusion

All experiments are done at 37 °C.

3.3.1 I/R Procedure

1. Incubate coverslip (*see* **Note 8**) in a separate container of Tyrode buffer for 15 min prior to ischemia.
2. Aspirate media in NMVMs and replace with 500 μL Tyrode buffer.
3. For ischemia:
   (a) Using forceps, place coverslip directly onto dish to cover NMVMs, avoid the formation of bubbles, and place dish back in incubator for 60 min.
4. For reperfusion:
   (a) Using forceps, gently remove coverslip and return dish to incubator for 60 min.
5. Following reperfusion, collect media and store in −80 °C to be used for further analysis and/or proceed to experimental readouts.

3.3.2 LDH Assay

1. Prepare reagents according to the manufacturer's instructions.
2. Put NMVMs through I/R procedure described above (Subheading 3.3.1).
3. Collect post-reperfusion media.
4. Transfer 50 μL of collected post-reperfusion media to a 96-well flat bottom plate.
5. Transfer 50 μL reaction mixture to each well.
6. Incubate at 37 °C for 30 min protected from light.

A

Absorbance at 490nm			
Sample 1	Sample 2	Sample 3	Media
4.042	3.963	2.935	0.365
3.869	4.035	2.82	0.366
3.506	3.817	2.948	0.39

Absorbance at 680nm			
Sample 1	Sample 2	Sample 3	Media
0.325	0.34	0.239	0.091
0.325	0.333	0.216	0.099
0.291	0.338	0.267	0.128

B

Subtract Absorbance at 680 from 490			
Sample 1	Sample 2	Sample 3	Media
3.717	3.623	2.696	0.274
3.544	3.702	2.604	0.267
3.215	3.479	2.681	0.262

Average Replicates			
Sample 1	Sample 2	Sample 3	Media
3.492	3.601	2.660	0.268

Subtract Media Readings		
Sample 1	Sample 2	Sample 3
4.042	3.963	2.935

C

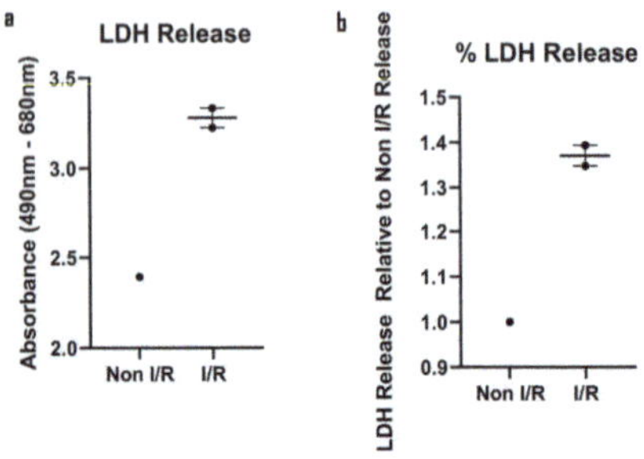

Fig. 1 (**A**) Raw absorbance values of a lactate dehydrogenase (LDH) assay read at 490 nm and 680 nm. Each sample was assayed in triplicate. (**B**) Values read at 680 nm are subtracted from values read at 490 nm for their corresponding wells. Values from control media is subtracted from sample values to remove background. (**C**) Quantification options as (a) absolute values or (b) normalized to non-ischemic samples (spontaneous LDH release)

7. Add 50 μL stop solution to each well, and then mix by gentle tapping.
8. Measure absorbance at 490 nm and 680 nm within 1–2 h.
9. Subtract 680 nm value from 490 nm value (Fig. 1).
10. Values can be plotted as absolute values or sample LDH release relative to spontaneous LDH release (Fig. 1; *see* **Note 9**).
11. *Optional: for LDH-positive control, transfer 50 uL 1× LDH-positive control to well plate.*

3.3.3 Mitochondrial Membrane Potential (MMP)

All experiments are done at 37 °C.

1. Load cells with 50 nM TMRM at 37 °C for 30 min prior to start of experiment.
2. Replace with 2.5 mL of fresh Tyrode buffer prior to imaging.
3. Cells were imaged and TMRM fluorescence was captured every 15 s for the duration of the protocol (Fig. 2):
   (a) 10 min to get baseline measurements.
   (b) 60 min of regional ischemia by placing a glass coverslip onto the dish.
   (c) 60 min of reperfusion by removal of the coverslip.

3.3.4 Image Analysis

1. Image series of the time course of ischemia/reperfusion experiments were analyzed using Fiji (https://imagej.net/Fiji/Downloads).
2. MMP response to I/R was analyzed at the cellular level by segmentation analysis on ImageJ (Fig. 3).
3. Segmentation analysis included a preprocessing step to align the images in the stack using a "StackReg" plugin [6].

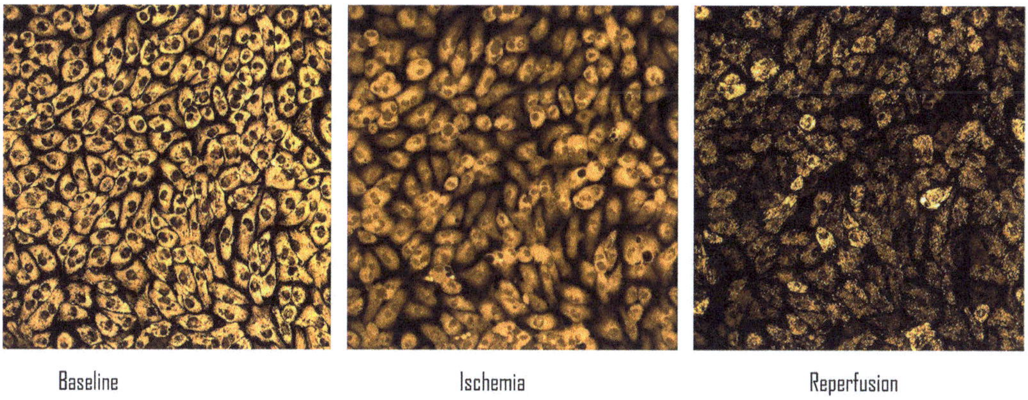

Fig. 2 Monolayer of neonatal mouse ventricular myocyte (NMVM) loaded with Tetramethyl rhodamine methyl ester (TMRM). Baseline shows TMRM fluorescence localized to energetically coupled mitochondria. Cells under ischemia show depolarized mitochondria where TMRM disperses into the cytoplasm exhibiting diffused distribution of TMRM fluorescence. At the end of reperfusion, damage due to ischemia is seen with certain cells completely losing their mitochondrial membrane potential

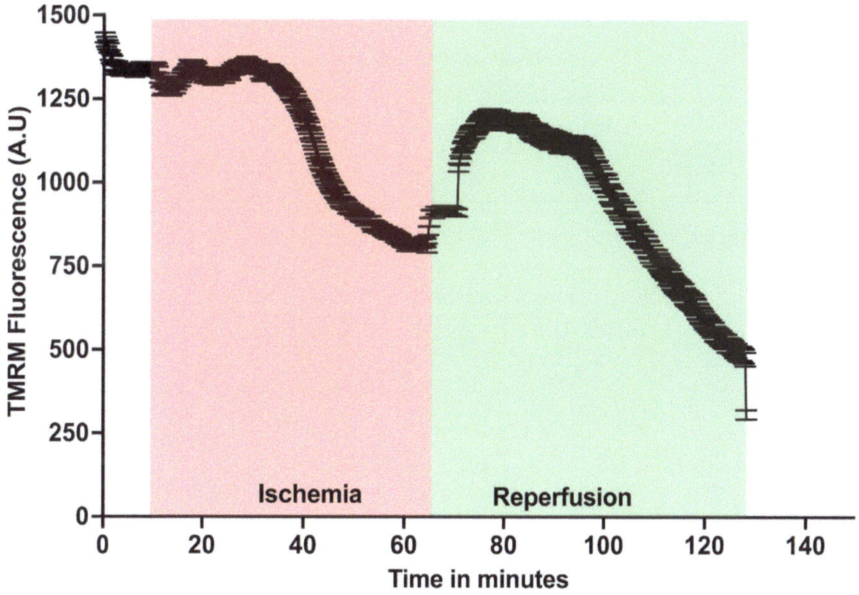

Fig. 3 Quantification of raw TMRM signals during ischemic and reperfusion periods using segmentation analysis. Representative TMRM trace of a single cardiomyocyte is shown above

4. Segmentation of each cell was done by applying a median filter (radius = 2) to the first image of the stack and then applying an auto local threshold (Niblack). All particles above the radius of 60 were included in the analysis.
5. Macros developed for image analysis to obtain TMRM fluorescence intensity for each cell over ischemia and reperfusion can be found at https://github.com/dashok1/MitoWave/tree/v1.0.2.

4 Notes

1. Vitamin B12 is light sensitive; solutions need to be prepared and stored in dark.
2. To avoid laser-induced damage, a neutral density filter of 10% was applied in the excitation path.
3. Fibronectin can also be dissolved in 1× PBS; however, some prefer water to avoid the possibility of salts interfering with plate adhesion/media components.
4. For a detailed protocol on cardiomyocyte isolation, see [7].
5. This rinses the blood out.
6. Ice-cold buffer is necessary to halt lysis and prevent over-digestion.
7. This flow-through contains unlabeled cells that are cardiomyocytes.
8. Coverslips handle can be made by using glass glue to adhere a small piece of aluminum foil, paperclip, or staple to the center of a standard glass cover slip.
9. Nonischemic control dishes of NMVMs should be used to capture "spontaneous LDH release."

Acknowledgments

This work was supported by the National Institutes of Health grant 1F31HL165820 (HG) and T32HL007227 (DA and OVE).

References

1. Jennings RB, Sommers HM, Smyth GA, Flack HA, Linn H (1960) Myocardial necrosis induced by temporary occlusion of a coronary artery in the dog. Arch Pathol 70:68–78
2. Pfeffer JM, Pfeffer MA, Braunwald E (1985) Influence of chronic captopril therapy on the infarcted left ventricle of the rat. Circ Res 57(1):84–95. https://doi.org/10.1161/01.res.57.1.84
3. Pfeffer MA, Pfeffer JM, Steinberg C, Finn P (1985) Survival after an experimental myocardial infarction: beneficial effects of long-term therapy with captopril. Circulation 72(2):406–412. https://doi.org/10.1161/01.cir.72.2.406
4. Tyers GF, Todd GJ, Neely JR, Waldhausen JA (1975) The mechanism of myocardial protection from ischemic arrest by intracoronary tetrodotoxin administration. J Thorac Cardiovasc Surg 69(2):190–195
5. Pitts KR, Toombs CF (2004) Coverslip hypoxia: a novel method for studying cardiac myocyte hypoxia and ischemia in vitro. Am J Phys Heart Circ Phys 287(4):H1801–H1812. https://doi.org/10.1152/ajpheart.00232.2004
6. Thévenaz P, Ruttimann UE, Unser M (1998) A pyramid approach to subpixel registration based on intensity. IEEE Trans Image Process 7(1):27–41. https://doi.org/10.1109/83.650848
7. Ehler E, Moore-Morris T, Lange S (2013) Isolation and culture of neonatal mouse cardiomyocytes. J Vis Exp 79. https://doi.org/10.3791/50154

Chapter 5

Induction on Insulin Resistance In Vitro

Eng Leng Saw

Abstract

Cellular model serves as a crucial preclinical research tool, providing essential insights into the mechanistic aspects of disease biology. Particularly in the study of chronic metabolic disorders such as type 2 diabetes mellitus and obesity, palmitate (a saturated fatty acid) is often used as a key inducer of insulin resistance in vitro. Within this chapter, I delineate procedures aimed at inducing insulin resistance in AC16 human cardiac-derived cells. The method involves the strategic application of heightened concentrations of palmitate and glucose to specifically target the AKT/GLUT-4 signaling pathway.

Key words Insulin resistance, Palmitate, Glucose, AC16 human cardiac-derived cells, AKT, GLUT-4

1 Introduction

Glucose transporter (GLUT)-4 plays a pivotal role in glucose metabolism as the primary insulin-responsive glucose uptake transporter in cardiac myocytes [1]. During the postprandial state, insulin activates phosphoinositide 3 kinase (PI3K)/protein kinase B (AKT) signaling, leading to the translocation of GLUT-4 to the plasma membrane to promote glucose uptake (reviewed in [2, 3]). However, in chronic metabolic disorders such as type 2 diabetes mellitus and obesity, GLUT-4 translocation and glucose uptake and utilization are impaired as the result of the development of insulin resistance in cardiac myocytes [4].

In the field of cardiovascular research, cellular models simulating insulin resistance are created through the application of heightened concentrations of glucose [5–7], palmitate [8, 9], insulin [10], or a combination of palmitate and insulin [11] to mimic the in vivo insulin-resistant state. Specifically, palmitate is recognized for its effect in inhibiting insulin-mediated glucose uptake by suppressing AKT activation [8, 11]. A previous study has established that a 16-h exposure to palmitate is adequate to reduce both basal and insulin-stimulated AKT activation in AC16 human

Dhananjie N. K. Chandrasekera and Rajesh Katare (eds.), *Cardiomyocytes: Methods and Protocols*, Methods in Molecular Biology, vol. 2894, https://doi.org/10.1007/978-1-0716-4342-6_5,

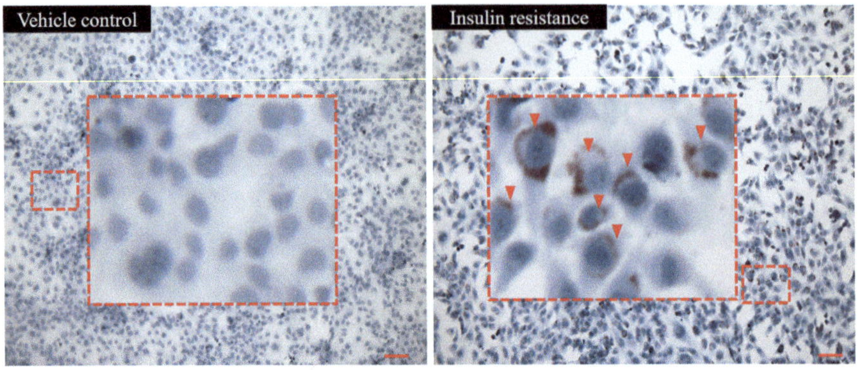

Fig. 1 Representative bright field images showing the ORO staining of vehicle control and insulin resistance AC16 cells after 48 hours of high glucose/palmitate treatment. Palmitate deposition stained by ORO appears in red color (indicated by red arrows) and hematoxylin-stained nuclei are in blue color. Scale bar = 100 μm

cardiac-derived cells. Yet, the impact of such an acute treatment duration on preventing GLUT-4 membrane translocation in AC16 cells remains uncertain [8]. Here, I demonstrate that 48-h exposure of high concentrations of palmitate and glucose induces insulin resistance in AC16 cells. Intracellular deposition of palmitate can be visualized by oil red o (ORO) staining (Fig. 1). On a molecular level, the impaired insulin-induced AKT activation and GLUT-4 translocation, which are both the important hallmarks of insulin resistance, are evident in these cells (Fig. 2).

In summary, this protocol outlines a methodology for establishing a cellular model of insulin resistance that recapitulates AKT/GLUT-4 signaling dysfunction observed in diabetic patients. Such a cellular model stands as a valuable research tool, offering insights into myocardial insulin resistance.

2 Materials

2.1 Culture of AC16 Human Cardiac-Derived Cells

1. Culture medium: Dulbecco's modified Eagle's medium (DMEM), 5% fetal bovine serum, and 1× antibiotic–antimycotic solution. Media stored at 4 °C.
2. TrypLE solution.
3. Sterile phosphate-buffered saline (PBS).
4. 75 cm^2 culture flask.
5. 60 mm cell culture dish.
6. 15 mm coverslips.
7. 24-well plates.
8. Palmitate/BSA complex solution: 10 mM sodium palmitate, 0.1 M NaOH, 10% (w/v) fatty acid-free bovine serum albumin.

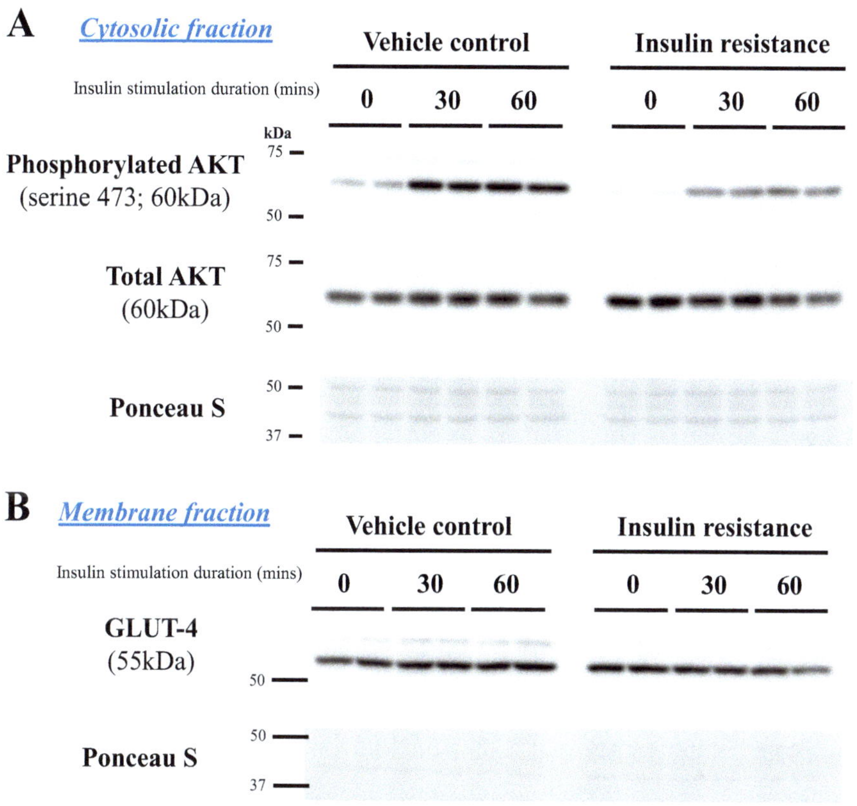

Fig. 2 Impaired AKT/GLUT-4 signaling in insulin resistance AC16 cells. Representative blots showing (**a**) decreased phosphorylation of AKT at serine 473 and (**b**) decreased membrane GLUT-4 protein expression in insulin resistance AC16 cells after 30 and 60 min insulin stimulation

(a) Initially, prepare a 100 mM sodium palmitate solution by dissolving sodium palmitate in 0.1 M sodium hydroxide solution at 70 °C (*see* **Note 1**). The solution should be aliquoted and stored at −20 °C. A 10% (w/v) fatty acid-free bovine serum albumin should be prepared, filtered, aliquoted, and stored at −20 °C. Finally, mix 100 mM sodium palmitate solution and 10% fatty acid-free BSA at 1:9 ratio at 55 °C (*see* **Note 2**). Solution is filtered, aliquoted, and stored at −20 °C.

9. Cell culture medium for induction of insulin resistance.

   (a) High glucose/palmitate culture medium: DMEM, 400 μM palmitate/BSA solution, 30.5 mM glucose, and 1× antibiotic–antimycotic solution. Culture medium stored at 4 °C.

   (b) Vehicle control culture medium: DMEM, 0.4% BSA solution, 5.5 mM glucose, 25 mM mannitol, and 1× antibiotic–antimycotic solution. Culture medium stored at 4 °C.

2.2 Oil Red O (ORO) Staining

1. 0.35% (w/v) ORO/isopropanol stock solution.
2. ORO working solution by mixing stock solution and distilled water at 6:4 ratio (*see* **Note 3**).
3. 60% isopropanol.
4. 4% paraformaldehyde (PFA) solution.
5. Mayer's hematoxylin solution.
6. Microscope glass slides.
7. Olympus BX61 Montaging light microscope.

2.3 Insulin Stimulation and Protein Sample Preparation

1. 500 mM human insulin solution.
2. Cell scrapers.
3. Mem-PER™ Plus Membrane Protein extraction kit (*see* **Note 4**).
4. Bio-Rad Bradford protein assay.
5. 6× Laemmli sample buffer: 12% sodium dodecyl sulfate (SDS), 60% glycerol, 30% β-mercaptoethanol, 0.012% bromophenol blue, 0.375 M Tris–HCl solution, pH 6.8.
6. Heat block.

2.4 Western Blot

1. Bio-Rad mini-PROTEAN® tetra vertical electrophoresis system.
2. Bio-Rad mini trans-blot® module includes holder cassettes, foam pads, and electrode assembly.
3. 1× running buffer: 25 mM Tris base, 192 mM glycine, and 0.1% SDS, pH 6.8.
4. 1× transfer buffer: 25 mM Tris base, 192 mM glycine, and 20% (v/v) methanol, pH 8.3.
5. 10% polyacrylamide gel.
6. Polyvinylidene difluoride (PVDF) membrane with 0.45 μM pore size.
7. Ponceau S solution: 0.1% (w/v) Ponceau S in 5% (v/v) acetic acid.
8. Blocking solution: 5% bovine serum albumin in TBS. Solution stored at 4 °C.
9. TBST buffer: 20 mM Tris base, 137 mM NaCl, 2.7 mM KCl, and 0.1% (v/v) Tween-20.
10. Plastic container.
11. Primary antibodies against phosphorylated AKT (serine 473; Cell Signaling, 9272), AKT (Cell Signaling, 9271), and GLUT-4 (NovusBio, BNP1–49533).
12. Anti-rabbit IgG-horseradish peroxidase (HRP)-conjugated secondary antibody.

13. Harsh stripping buffer: 20 mL 10% SDS, 12.5 mL 0.5 M Tris–HCl solution (pH 6.8), 0.8 mL β-mercaptoethanol, 67.5 mL distilled water.
14. Bio-Rad Clarity™ western ECL substrates.
15. Syngene Pxi imaging system.

3 Methods

3.1 Cell Culture

1. Maintain AC16 cells in a 75 cm^2 flask with culture medium at 37 °C and 5% CO_2. Replace medium every 2 days.
2. Upon reaching 90–100% confluency, detach cells from the flask using TrypLE solution. Collect and centrifuge the cellular suspension at 300× *g* for 5 min to pellet the cells.
3. Discard the supernatant and resuspend the cell pellet in fresh culture medium.
4. Seed the cells in a 24-well plate with 15 mm cover slip in each well or 60 mm cell culture dish for ORO staining and Western blot analysis, respectively.

3.2 ORO Staining

1. Seed AC16 cells on a coverslip in a 24-well plate at a density of 0.6×10^5 cells/cm^2 (*see* **Note 5**). This density ensures approximately 70% confluency after overnight attachment.
2. Replace the medium with either high glucose/palmitate culture medium or vehicle control culture medium and incubate for 48 h.
3. Remove the cell culture media and wash cells with sterile PBS solution. Fix cells with 4% PFA solution for 15 min at room temperature. Remove the 4% PFA solution and wash cells with PBS solution three times for 5 min each.
4. Treat cells with 60% isopropanol three times for 1 min each.
5. Incubate cells with freshly prepared ORO working solution for 1 h at room temperature.
6. Remove ORO working solution and incubate cells with 60% isopropanol for 5 min. Rinse cells with distilled water at least three times for 3 min each (*see* **Note 6**).
7. Incubate cells with Mayer's hematoxylin solution for 10 min.
8. Wash cells with distilled water three times for 3 min each.
9. Carefully remove the coverslip from the 24-well plate and mount it on a microscope slide using mounting medium. Allow the slide to dry overnight.
10. View the stained cells under a light microscope to assess palmitate uptake (Fig. 1).

3.3 Insulin Stimulation and Protein Sample Preparation

1. Seed AC16 cells on 60 mm culture dish at a density of 0.6×10^5 cells/cm^2.
2. Replace the medium with either high glucose/palmitate culture medium or vehicle control culture medium and incubate for 48 h.
3. Add 500 mM human insulin and incubate for 30 and 60 min. Cells without insulin stimulation serve as the negative control.
4. Harvest cells using cell scraper. Utilize the Mem-PER™ Plus Membrane Protein extraction kit following the manufacturer's instruction to separate cytosolic- and membrane-enriched proteins.
5. Quantify the protein sample concentration using Bio-Rad Bradford protein assay as per manufacturer's instruction.
6. Dilute protein samples with 6× Laemmli buffer and denature at 95 °C for 5 min using a heat block.
7. Aliquot protein samples and store at −80 °C.

3.4 Western Blot

1. Load 20 μg of cytosolic- and membrane-enriched proteins onto 10% polyacrylamide gels, respectively. Perform electrophoresis at 150 V in 1× running buffer until the dye front reaches the bottom of the gel.
2. Transfer proteins from the gel to a PVDF membrane in 1× transfer buffer using the Bio-Rad mini trans-blot® module at 110 V for 90 min.
3. Stain the PVDF membrane with Ponceau S solution for 1 min. Wash the membrane with distilled water for 1 min and capture an image.
4. Wash PVDF membrane with TBST solution five to ten times to completely remove Ponceau S staining.
5. Block the PVDF membrane with a blocking solution for 1 h at room temperature.
6. Dilute primary antibody in the blocking solution (*see* **Note 7**).
7. Incubate the PVDF membrane with the primary antibody solution overnight.
8. Following overnight incubation, wash the PVDF membrane with TBST solution three times for 5 min.
9. Dilute secondary antibody in the blocking solution (*see* **Note 7**). Incubate the membrane with secondary antibody solution for 1 h at room temperature.
10. Wash the PVDF membrane with TBST solution three times for 5 min.

11. Incubate the membrane with ECL substrates following the manufacturer's instruction. Image the membrane using an imager (Fig. 2).
12. After detecting phosphorylated AKT expression, strip the membrane with a strong stripping buffer at 50 °C for 30 min followed by extensive wash with TBST solution five to ten times (*see* **Note 8**).
13. Repeat **steps 5–11** to detect total AKT expression (*see* **Note 9**; Fig. 2).

4 Notes

1. Use a water bath set at 70 °C to dissolve sodium palmitate. Gently swirl to ensure efficient dissolution.
2. Pre-heat an aliquot of 100 mM sodium palmitate solution on a heat block and immediately mix it with 10% fatty acid-free bovine serum albumin. Perform this step using a heat block.
3. Prepare ORO working solution freshly for optimal staining result.
4. For efficient protein isolation, it is essential to supplement the permeabilization buffer and solubilization buffer obtained from the Mem-PER™ Plus Membrane Protein extraction kit with 1× cOmplete™ protease inhibitor cocktail, 1× PhosSTOP™ phosphatase inhibitor cocktail, and 100 mM phenylmethanesulfonyl fluoride (PMSF).
5. The recommended seeding density of 0.6×10^5 cells/cm^2 accounts for potential cell death/loss after 48 h of high glucose/palmitate treatment. Avoid using a seeding density lower than this value.
6. To minimize background, perform an extensive wash with distilled water after staining procedures.
7. Dilute antibodies as follows: anti-phosphorylated AKT antibody (serine 473), 1:1000; anti-GLUT-4 antibody, 1:2500; anti-rabbit IgG-HRP-conjugated secondary antibody, 1:5000.
8. Due to the presence of β-mercaptoethanol in the stripping buffer, ensure an extensive wash to completely remove any residual traces.
9. Dilute antibodies as follows: anti-AKT antibody, 1:1000; anti-rabbit IgG-HRP-conjugated secondary antibody, 1:5000.

Acknowledgements

The research detailed in this chapter was conducted at the Department of Physiology, University of Otago, with support from the Royal Society of New Zealand Catalyst Seed Funding (18-UOO-011-CSG), Lottery Health research funding (R-LHR-2020-128280), and the University of Otago Research Grant. E.L.S. was supported by the University of Otago Doctoral Scholarship, Elizabeth Jean Trotter Postgraduate Research Travelling Scholarship in Biomedical Sciences, and research funding from the Department of Physiology. E.L.S. is currently affiliated with Boston University and supported by NHLBI of the National Institutes of Health under award RO1HL145985 (to Dr. Flora Sam) and Whitaker Cardiovascular Institute Pilot Grant awards.

References

1. Fukumoto H, Kayano T, Buse JB, Edwards Y, Pilch PF, Bell GI, Seino S (1989) Cloning and characterization of the major insulin-responsive glucose transporter expressed in human skeletal muscle and other insulin-responsive tissues. J Biol Chem 264(14): 7776–7779
2. Montessuit C, Lerch R (2013) Regulation and dysregulation of glucose transport in cardiomyocytes. Biochim Biophys Acta 1833(4): 848–856. https://doi.org/10.1016/j.bbamcr.2012.08.009
3. Shao D, Tian R (2015) Glucose transporters in cardiac metabolism and hypertrophy. Compr Physiol 6(1):331–351. https://doi.org/10.1002/cphy.c150016
4. Freeman AM, Acevedo LA, Pennings N (2024) Insulin resistance. Treasure Island (FL): StatPearls Publishing. https://www.ncbi.nlm.nih.gov/books/NBK507839/
5. Davidoff AJ, Davidson MB, Carmody MW, Davis ME, Ren J (2004) Diabetic cardiomyocyte dysfunction and myocyte insulin resistance: role of glucose-induced PKC activity. Mol Cell Biochem 262(1–2):155–163
6. Rawal S, Nagesh PT, Coffey S, Van Hout I, Galvin IF, Bunton RW, Davis P, Williams MJA, Katare R (2019) Early dysregulation of cardiac-specific microRNA-208a is linked to maladaptive cardiac remodelling in diabetic myocardium. Cardiovasc Diabetol 18(1):13–13. https://doi.org/10.1186/s12933-019-0814-4
7. Rawal S, Munasinghe PE, Shindikar A, Paulin J, Cameron V, Manning P, Williams MJA, Jones GT, Bunton R, Galvin I, Katare R (2017) Down-regulation of proangiogenic microRNA-126 and microRNA-132 are early modulators of diabetic cardiac microangiopathy. Cardiovasc Res 113(1):90–101. https://doi.org/10.1093/cvr/cvw235
8. Chokshi A, Drosatos K, Cheema FH, Ji R, Khawaja T, Yu S, Kato T, Khan R, Takayama H, Knoll R, Milting H, Chung CS, Jorde U, Naka Y, Mancini DM, Goldberg IJ, Schulze PC (2012) Ventricular assist device implantation corrects myocardial lipotoxicity, reverses insulin resistance, and normalizes cardiac metabolism in patients with advanced heart failure. Circulation 125(23): 2844–2853. https://doi.org/10.1161/circulationaha.111.060889
9. Tsuchiya Y, Hatakeyama H, Emoto N, Wagatsuma F, Matsushita S, Kanzaki M (2010) Palmitate-induced down-regulation of sortilin and impaired GLUT4 trafficking in C2C12 myotubes. J Biol Chem 285(45): 34371–34381. https://doi.org/10.1074/jbc.M110.128520
10. Bertrand L, Ginion A, Beauloye C, Hebert AD, Guigas B, Hue L, Vanoverschelde JL (2006) AMPK activation restores the stimulation of glucose uptake in an in vitro model of insulin-resistant cardiomyocytes via the activation of protein kinase B. Am J Physiol Heart Circ Physiol 291(1):H239–H250. https://doi.org/10.1152/ajpheart.01269.2005

11. Schwenk RW, Angin Y, Steinbusch LKM, Dirkx E, Hoebers N, Coumans WA, Bonen A, Broers JLV, van Eys GJJM, Glatz JFC, Luiken JJFP (2012) Overexpression of vesicle-associated membrane protein (VAMP) 3, but not VAMP2, protects glucose transporter (GLUT) 4 protein translocation in an in vitro model of cardiac insulin resistance. J Biol Chem 287(44):37530–37539. https://doi.org/10.1074/jbc.M112.363630

Chapter 6

Preparation of Human Atrial Trabeculae for Ex Vivo Analysis of Human Myocardial Function

Hamish M. Aitken-Buck, Kyra T. Bingham, and Regis R. Lamberts

Abstract

Human myocardial function can be investigated in the laboratory using human atrial trabeculae. These multicellular preparations provide a translatable model for assessing the ex vivo contractility, electrophysiology, and ionic and metabolic underpinnings of human cardiac muscle. Here, we detail the materials and methods required to determine the baseline function of a human atrial trabecula, from dissection to stimulation. This method is also adaptable for additional non-human myocardial applications.

Key words Human atrial trabeculae, Human myocardium, Contractility, Method

1 Introduction

Human atrial trabeculae are an invaluable multicellular preparation for the study of human myocardial function. Since the 1980s [1, 2], researchers have used atrial trabeculae to investigate myocardial contractility and electrophysiology, with the findings carrying translatability afforded to human tissues. In contemporary cardiovascular research, atrial trabeculae are also commonly used to study the nuances of ionic and metabolic homeostasis in the heart [3–5] and the effectiveness of drugs [6, 7]. Here, we detail the method for successfully dissecting, mounting, and stimulating a human atrial trabecula. We also outline standard methods for data collection and analysis. This method provides the foundation for other physiological measurements from human myocardial trabecula (*see* **Note 1**).

2 Materials

2.1 Solutions

Prepare all solutions fresh on the day of experimentation using ultrapure water and analytical grade reagents. Stock solutions of

Dhananjie N. K. Chandrasekera and Rajesh Katare (eds.), *Cardiomyocytes: Methods and Protocols*, Methods in Molecular Biology, vol. 2894, https://doi.org/10.1007/978-1-0716-4342-6_6,

select reagents can be prepared in advance. However, $NaHCO_3^-$ and glucose should be added on the day of use to prevent $CaCO_3$ precipitation and microorganism growth, respectively. For this protocol, solutions are based on Krebs–Henseleit buffer formulations (*see* **Note 2**).

1. Cardioplegia solution composition: 118.5 mM NaCl, 4.5 KCl, 1.0 mM $MgCl_26H_2O$, 0.33 mM NaH_2PO_4, 25.0 mM $NaHCO_3$, 0.25 mM $CaCl_2$, 11.0 mM glucose, 25.0 mM 2,3-butanedione monoxime (BDM). Oxygenated with carbogen (95% O_2:5% CO_2), pH 7.4, ice-cold (*see* **Note 3**).
2. Tissue bath superfusion solution composition: 118.5 mM NaCl, 4.5 mM KCl, 1.0 mM $MgCl_26H_2O$, 0.33 mM NaH_2PO_4, 25.0 mM $NaHCO_3$, 0.25–1.5 mM $CaCl_2$, 11.0 mM glucose. Oxygenated with carbogen (95% O_2:5% CO_2), pH 7.4, 37 °C.

2.2 Trabecula Microdissection Setup

A typical trabecula microdissection setup is shown in Fig. 1.

1. Microdissection plate: Walled plated with cushioned surface penetrable to fine-point pins. Must be cleanable, with replenishable volume of 5–10 mL and bracing for a carbogen infusion line.

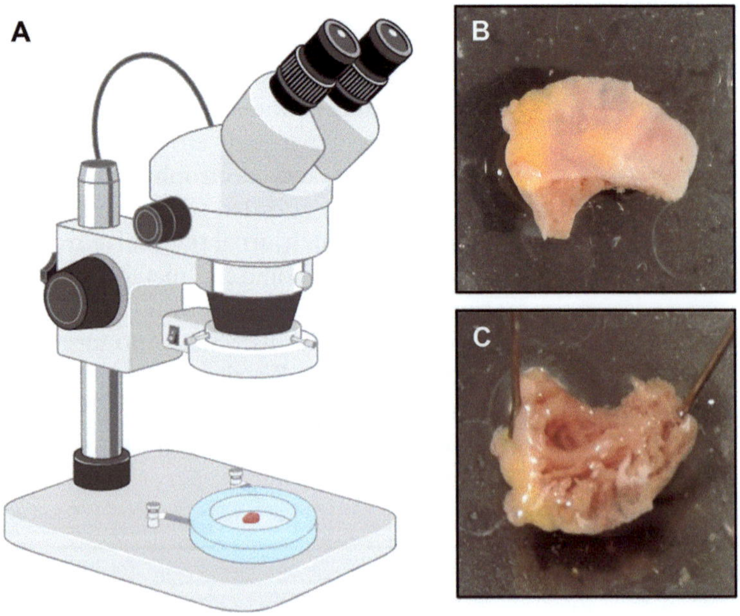

Fig. 1 Human right atrial appendage and trabecula dissection. (**a**), Schematic representation of stereoscope with intact human atrial appendage biopsy housed in the walled microdissection plate. Photographs of a human right atrial appendage biopsy are shown in (**b**) and (**c**). In (**b**), the biopsy is intact with the endocardial surface obscured by the epicardium. In (**c**), the biopsy has been carefully cut and opened to expose the endocardial surface, which contains trabeculae

2. Stereoscope: Stereoscope with removable ocular eyepiece, mounted above microdissection plate.
3. Light source: Lamp with adjustable light intensity and light position.
4. Microdissection tools: Fine-tip forceps (×2), medium-tip microdissection scissors, fine-tip microdissection scissors. All sterilized with ultrasonication.

2.3 Trabecula Bath System

A typical trabecula bath and stimulation system is shown in Fig. 2 (also *see* **Note 4**).

1. Horizontal tissue bath: 2.5 mL volume, minimal volume 0.5 mL. We use the SI-H Horizontal Tissue Bath (SI Heidelberg, World Precision Instruments, Inc.). Bath is fitted with in-house custom-made horizontal platinum electrodes for electric field stimulation.
2. Removable mounting slide: Plastic slide with small divot for temporary placement of dissected trabeculae. Can be removed after trabecula is mounted.

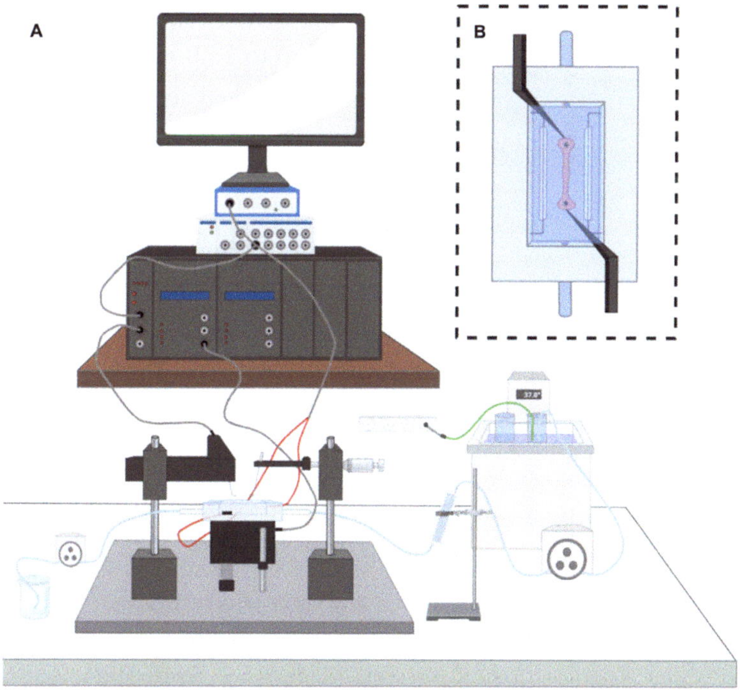

Fig. 2 Human atrial trabecula horizontal bath system. (**a**), Schematic representation of a standard trabecula horizontal tissue bath and supporting components. (**b**) (inset), horizontal tissue bath viewed from above, with visualization of trabecula mounting on transducer hooks. Note, the trabecula and bath components in (**b**) are not to scale: a human trabecula will be significantly smaller in length and diameter

3. Trabecula mount: Pointed hook tissue mount. Connected to appropriate force transducer (*see* **Note 5**).
4. Muscle length manipulator: Spindle-type micromanipulator connected to trabecula mount via fixed arm. Must have appropriate resolution (0.1 mm). Can rely on manual readout, but digital is preferred.
5. Force transducer: With fitted muscle-mounting fine-point hook. Should have appropriate sensitivity and range for capturing raw force produced by trabecula contraction (for human trabeculae: 0–20 mN).
6. Electric field stimulator: Constant-current (20–2000 mA) or constant-voltage (0.5–64 V) capable electrical stimulator. Typical biphasic stimulus specifications of 0.05–999 Hz frequency and 10 μs–99 s duration (*see* **Note 6**).
7. Water bath: Recirculating water bath with 37 °C capacity.
8. Bath temperature controller: Programmed to 37 °C set point. Built into most commercial horizontal tissue bath.
9. Oxygenation and pH balancing: Carbogen gas (95% O_2:5% CO_2) with multiple outflow lines and taps.
10. Solution pumps: 2× peristalsis pumps (1× inflow, 1× outflow) capable of up to 15.0 mL/min flow rate.
11. Solution tubing and accessories (*see* **Note 7**):
    (a) Peristaltic pump silicon tubing with stops compatible with the peristaltic pump. Tubing with 2.4 mm internal diameter allows up to 15.0 mL/min flow rate.
    (b) Silicon tubing of variable calibre, internal diameter 3.1 mm, cut to appropriate lengths to facilitate solution delivery and removal, and recirculation (if desired, *see* **Note 8**).
    (c) Tubing adapters and (if necessary) three-way valves to connect tubing types to each other and to tissue bath inlet and outlet.
    (d) Glass-jacketed perfusion coil. Enables conductive heat transfer during transit of solution from water bath to tissue bath. Requires inlet and outlet for solution flow and inlet and outlet for heated water flow.
12. Data acquisition: Multichannel data acquisition system hardware and software. Must allow real-time data acquisition with time synchronization between channels, filtering and noise reduction, and live parameter derivation from raw signal.
13. Structural support: Configuration of the bath system components can require support from magnetic and nonmagnetic stands and clamps of various sizes.

3 Methods

3.1 Solution Preparation and Tissue Collection

- Prepare 100 mL of cardioplegia solution, place on ice, and oxygenate with carbogen for at least 30 min prior to collection of atrial appendage biopsy.
- At the same time, prepare the tissue bath superfusion solution (0.25 mM $CaCl_2$) in a graduated cylinder or other receptacle with sufficient volume. Place in the circulating water bath at 37 ° C and oxygenate with carbogen (*see* **Note 9**). Cover the top of the open-ended solution receptacle with parafilm.
- Collect atrial appendage (*see* **Note 10**) in ~50 mL of the pre-oxygenated and chilled cardioplegia solution. Reserve the remaining ~50 mL for trabecula dissection in the laboratory.

3.2 Trabecula Microdissection

1. Remove the atrial appendage from the cardioplegia solution using fine-tip forceps and place into a dissection stage filled with fresh ice-cold cardioplegia solution that is continuously oxygenated with carbogen (Fig. 1b).
2. Carefully orientate the atrial appendage so the endocardial surface can be seen. Using sterile pins, secure the atrial appendage to the dissection stage (Fig. 1c). Make small incisions to open expose the endocardial surface if necessary.
3. Under the stereoscope, identify trabeculae that are non-branching, not adhered to the endocardial surface along the longitudinal axis, and can be easily accessed by microdissection using forceps and scissors. Use a micrometer eyepiece to refine candidate trabeculae to only those with sufficiently small diameter (preferably <0.2 mm; *see* **Note 11**).
4. Without stretching the trabecula, carefully cut a small piece of appendage at both ends of the trabecula, roughly twice the three-dimensional area of the trabecula. Once cut, the trabecula should be liberated from the appendage ready for mounting (*see* **Note 12**).

3.3 Trabecula Mounting

1. Begin superfusion of the trabecula tissue bath with warmed and oxygenated superfusion solution. Note this superfusion solution contains 0.25 mM $CaCl_2$.
2. Using a Pasteur pipette, transfer the dissected trabecula and ~ 3–4 mL of cardioplegia solution to the removable mounting slide on the tissue bath system.
3. Wind the micromanipulator dial, so the force transducer hooks or baskets are closer together than the length of the relaxed trabecula. This is to avoid stretching the trabecula.

4. Orientate the removable mounting slide containing the trabecula and cardioplegia solution underneath the force transducer hooks. Lower the hooks into the cardioplegia solution.
5. Carefully align the edges of the trabecula above the force transducer hooks with fine-point forceps. Apply gentle pressure to the dissected pieces of appendage at each end of the trabecula to mount it on the force transducer hooks (*see* **Note 13**). Make sure the trabecula is aligned at 180° with the force transducer. Do not touch the contractile region of the trabecula at any stage.

3.4 Equilibrating, Stimulating, and Stretching the Trabecula

1. Carefully lower the mounted trabecula and force transducer hooks into the tissue bath containing pre-warmed and oxygenated superfusion solution. The trabecula should be submerged in superfusion solution and positioned evenly between the platinum recording electrodes.
2. Begin recording the raw force output from the trabecula and allow it to equilibrate in the superfusion solution for at least 30 min.
3. When equilibrated, begin 1 Hz (60 beats per minute) electrical field stimulation (5 ms rectangular pulse) at minimal voltage or current (depending on stimulation system). Increase stimulus intensity in ~10% increments until an inducible 1 Hz contraction is observable (*see* **Note 14**).
4. Once a stimulated contraction has been achieved, increase the $CaCl_2$ concentration in 0.25 mM increments over a ~ 20–30-min period to a final concentration of 1.0–1.8 mM (depending on the required experimental concentration).
5. Once at the final $CaCl_2$ concentration, resume the incremental increases in electrical stimulus intensity until an increase in intensity is no longer accompanied by an increase in contraction force (i.e., maximal voltage/current). At this point, increase the stimulus intensity by 10–15% to achieve a supramaximal intensity.
6. Using the micromanipulator, gradually increase the trabecula length in ~0.1–0.2 μm increments until an increase in length is no longer accompanied by an increase in contraction force (this approximates 2.1–2.2 μm sarcomere length and this muscle length is often referred to as L_{max}) [8]. Allow the passive stress to return to pre-stretch level before initiating the next stretch. Once at maximal stretch, reduce the trabecula length to 95% of the maximum muscle length (95% L_{max}).
7. The trabecula should now be contracting at a programmed frequency with physiological availability of extracellular Ca^{2+} and at ideal sarcomere length. This is the baseline functional characteristics of the trabecula. Proceed with additional experimental protocol if required (*see* **Note 15**).

3.5 Data Analysis

1. Derivation of common parameters (*see* Fig. 3a): A contracting trabecula will yield a *raw isometric force trace* with a measurable upward deflection in isometric force during contraction and a downward deflection from maximal isometric force during relaxation. Several technical and functional parameters can be derived from this raw isometric force trace. Commonly this includes (but not limited to) the following:
   (a) *Stimulus artifact:* If integrated with the software, the time-point of individual electrical stimulation events can be analyzed. Useful for post hoc determination of programmed stimulation frequency and for temporal alignment of stimulus and contractility phases.
   (b) *Contraction frequency:* Derived from *raw force trace* as a cyclic measurement of contraction frequency (*see* **Note 16**).
   (c) *Stress (normalized isometric force, mN/mm^2):* Calculated by normalization of *raw force trace* at each time-point to trabecula cross-sectional area (*see* **Note 17**).
   (d) *Active stress:* Derived from *stress* trace as amplitude of contraction relative to baseline. In other words, the amount of stress generated during contraction.
   (e) *Diastolic (passive) stress:* Derived from *stress* trace as the minimum value in each contraction–relaxation cycle.
2. Analyzing contraction peak parameters (*see* Fig. 3b): Besides the absolute isometric force and normalized stress, many other parameters can be determined from off-line analysis of trabecula functional data. Common single peak contraction and relaxation parameters are presented in Table 1. Analysis of trabecula functional parameters should be performed across several full contraction cycles for each period of interest (e.g., baseline function, after drug treatment). Typically, the final 30–60 s of each period is used (*see* **Note 18**).

4 Notes

1. Additional measurements include the following (but are not limited to):
   (a) *Electrophysiology:* Electrophysiological recording of human myocardial trabecula is a common additional (if not primary) measurement for many research groups [6, 7]. Atrial action potentials are recorded with glass micropipette intracellular electrodes (10–50 MΩ resistance) filled with KCl (3 M). Parameters commonly

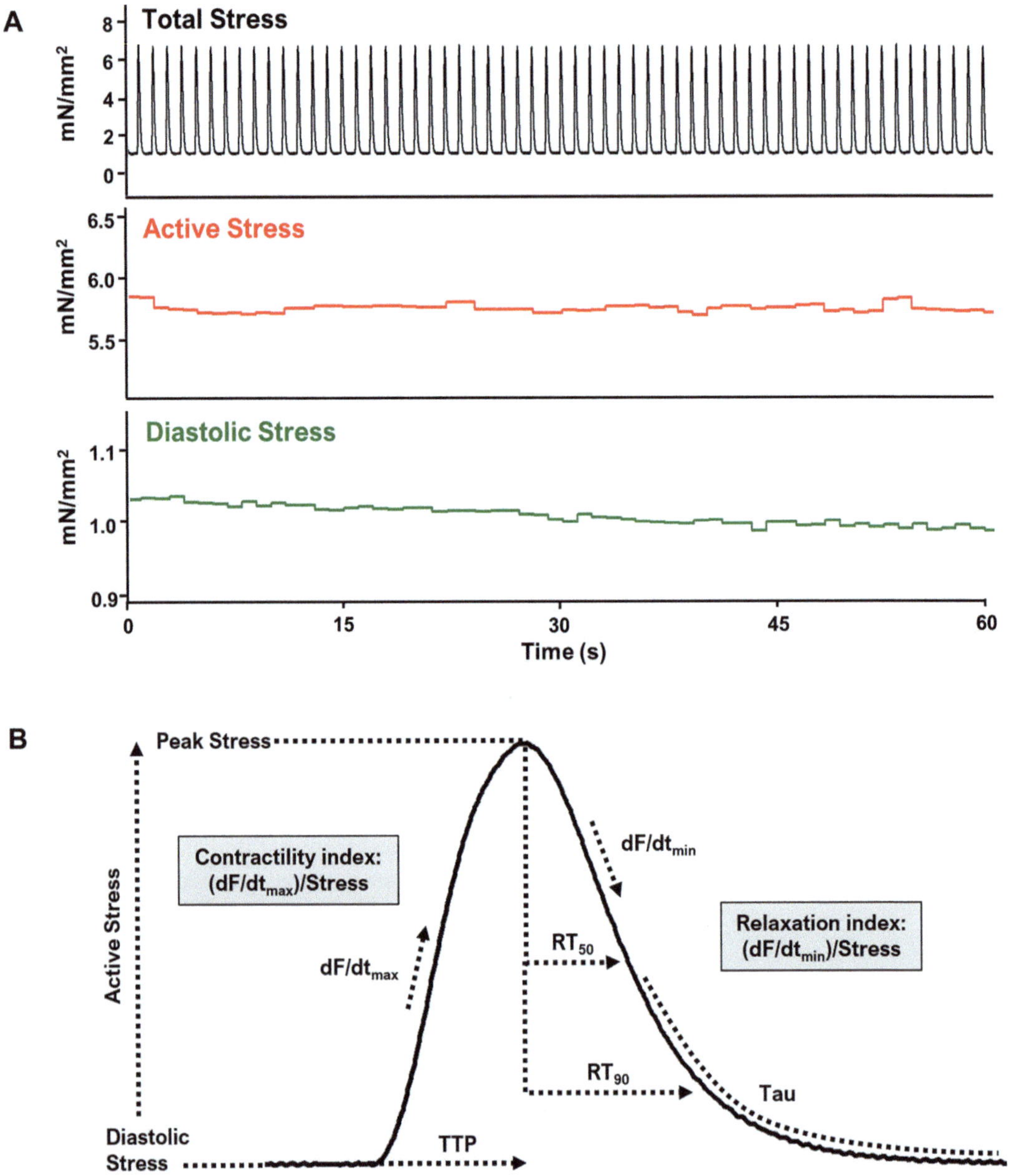

Fig. 3 Functional recording of human atrial trabecula and single contraction analysis parameters. (**a**), 60-s functional recording from a single human atrial trabecula. Total stress (normalized to trabecula cross-sectional area, mN/mm^2) is shown in the top channel (black). Active (derivation shown in **b**) and diastolic stresses derived from total stress channel are shown in the red and green channels, respectively. (**b**), Derivation of common single peak parameters. TTP = time to peak; dF/dt_{max} = maximal slope of contraction; dF/dt_{min} = maximal slope of relaxation; RT_{50} = time to 50% relaxation from peak; RT_{90} = time to 90% relaxation from peak

Table 1
Common functional parameters derived from a single contraction–relaxation cycle of a human atrial trabecula. Raw isometric force parameters are normalized to index chosen by the author; raw trabecula force has been normalized to trabecula cross-sectional area. RT = relaxation time

Parameter	Unit	Definition
Contraction parameters		
Active stress	mN/mm^2	Normalized isometric force generated during contraction phase
Time to peak	Ms	Time from onset of contraction to maximal force
dF/dt_{max}	$mN/mm^2/s$	Maximal slope (velocity) of contraction upstroke
Contractility index	1/s	Maximal slope of contraction divided by active force
Relaxation parameters		
RT_{50}	Ms	Time from maximal stress to 50% relaxation
RT_{90}	Ms	Time from maximal stress to 90% relaxation
dF/dt_{min}	$mN/mm^2/s$	Maximal slope (velocity) of relaxation downstroke
Tau	Ms	Exponential time constant of relaxation
Relaxation index	1/s	Maximal slope of relaxation divided by active stress

measured include the amplitude, duration, upstroke velocity, and refractory periods of action potentials, as well as resting membrane potential. Can be recorded in parallel with trabecula force measurement.

(b) *Biofluorometry:* A range of fluorescent molecular indicators can be loaded into a trabecula to gain insight into the physiology of the contracting myocardium. This can include indicators for changes in membrane potential, ATPase activity (and thus metabolism products), and intracellular ions [4], most commonly Ca^{2+} [3, 9].

2. Similar success can be achieved using MOPS-(3-(N-morpholino) propanesulfonic acid), HEPES-(4-(2-hydroxyethyl)-1-piperazineethanesulfonic acid), or HCO_3^--based solutions adapted from Ringer (Tyrode) formulations for trabecula cardioplegia and superfusion. MOPS- and HEPES-based cardioplegia solutions do not rely on oxygenation with carbogen for pH maintenance. Regardless of the source formulation and composition stoichiometry, trabecula superfusion solution requires the core components of Na^+ ions (excitability and contractility), Cl^- ions (isotonicity), K^+ ions (muscle relaxation), Ca^{2+} and Mg^{2+} ions (contraction), $NaHCO_3^-$ and/or NaH_2PO_4 (pH buffering), and glucose or pyruvate (metabolism).

3. The viability of human atrial trabeculae collected during surgery is extended by arresting metabolic and contractile processes during transit from the surgical theatre to the laboratory. This is commonly achieved by including myosin ATPase inhibitor, BDM, in ice-cold low-Ca^{2+} cardioplegia solution [10].
4. It is advantageous to have two (or more) identical trabecula bath systems that can be operated in parallel. Logistically, it allows more trabeculae to be tested from each precious atrial appendage biopsy, increasing the likelihood of identifying a viable trabecula from each tissue donor. It is important to note that not all trabeculae from the same appendage will successfully contract. Scientifically, having parallel systems allows for different experimental protocols to be performed on trabecula from the same patient, which can limit the effect of inter-patient variability when comparing interventions.
5. Trabeculae can also be successfully mounted using other commercially available tissue mounts, including tweezer and basket mounts.
6. Most commercially available electrical stimulators can be integrated with a computer, which, using specific software, allows for control of stimulus triggering and programming of stimulus patterns. The latter is ideal for delivering periods of uniform stimuli, such as the delivery of arrhythmia-initiating trains of high-frequency pulses.
7. It is useful to determine the dead space volume of the tubing (i.e., volume between KHB reservoir and tissue bath) and the time required for solution delivery from the reservoir to the tissue bath at different pump speeds. This is especially important if exact timings are required for exposure to different solutions: the delivery time can be accounted for in exposure time.
8. The tubing system can be configured to empty into the solution reservoir and allow solution recirculation. Alternatively, the outflow tubing can be emptied into a waste receptacle to have one-way circulation. The latter is useful if the experiment requires determination of uptake of a superfusion factor by the trabecula or the secretion of a factor into the superfusion solution by the trabecula. Moreover, if the experimental protocol is of significant duration, prolonged solution recirculation can contribute to trabecula deterioration due to the accumulation of waste products and depletion of finite solution components.
9. Oxygenation with carbogen is essential to set the pH of the KHB solution to 7.4. The pH of the KHB solution should be checked prior to commencing a trabecula experiment.

10. It is important to carefully consider the characteristics of the patients from whom the right atrial appendage has been procured. Trabecula contractility, electrophysiology, and drug responsiveness are known to be influenced to various degrees by patient characteristics, including female sex, body mass index, hypertension and hyperlipidemia diagnoses, left ventricular ejection fraction and end-diastolic volume, and medications such as β-blockers [11, 12]. Therefore, care should be taken to ensure to control for these variables when designing trabecula experiments, especially if a single patient characteristic defines comparison groups (i.e., a disease group vs. non-diseased group).
11. The demands of a trabecula are dependent on diffusion of oxygen and nutrients. Hence, muscle cross-sectional area is a key determinant of the function and viability and thus success of a human atrial trabecula experiment. Evidence from animal and human studies suggests that trabecula function can be negatively affected if trabecula diameter exceeds 0.15–0.2 mm (assuming working experiment temperature of 37 °C) [13, 14]. Therefore, trabeculae with diameters less than this critical value should be used to prevent the formation of a hypoxic/anoxic core within the trabecula during the experiment.
12. Multicellular cardiac preparations such as human atrial trabeculae are highly sensitive to overstretching. To improve experimental success rate, never overstretch the trabecula. A helpful tip to prevent overstretching is to never touch the atrial appendage or a trabecula with microdissection tools without looking under the stereoscope at what you are doing.
13. Alternatively, mounting sites can be prepared on each end of the trabecula while in the dissection dish using a sterile fine-tip pin. In our experience, fibrotic appendages can be difficult to pierce, resulting in accidental damage to the trabecula through overstretching or contact with the contractile region when mounting onto the hooks of the force transducer. Preparing holes for the force transducer hooks before mounting can reduce the chances of this happening and increase the likelihood of the trabecula remaining viable.
14. In our experience, a viable human trabecula can take several minutes to respond to the initiation of the electrical stimulus. This contrasts with viable multicellular myocardial preparations from animal models that typically respond instantly to electrical stimulus. If the human atrial trabecula does not contract immediately, wait several minutes before increasing the stimulus intensity.

15. Downstream applications can include the following (but are not limited to):
   (a) *Contractility and relaxation effects:* Contractility (inotropic) and relaxation (lusitropic) effects of many factors can be tested using this preparation [3, 6, 15]. This includes the effect of drug infusion, a change in superfusate nutrient or ion composition [16], a temperature change, or a change in trabecula (sarcomere) length [4].
   (b) *Arrhythmia susceptibility:* Unstimulated (i.e., arrhythmic) contractions can be acutely induced using adrenergic agonists such as isoproterenol (30–100 nM) alone or in conjunction with high extracellular Ca^{2+} (2–5 mM) [6, 15, 17]. Arrhythmia-like contractions can manifest as distinct spontaneous contractions (i.e., in the prolonged absence of electrical stimulation) or premature or delayed extra-contractions (during interstimulation period). Bursts (also called "trains") of higher-frequency (2–3 Hz) electrical stimulation lasting 10–15 s can also trigger arrhythmia-like contractions [18]. Susceptibility to burst-induced arrhythmias is increased if extracellular Ca^{2+} is also increased. Arrhythmia susceptibility is commonly quantified as a binary outcome of presence or absence of arrhythmias [6, 17, 19], by researcher-defined arrhythmia severity scores, or number of arrhythmic events [17].
   (c) *Stress–frequency relationship:* Used to indirectly assess myofilament Ca^{2+} sensitivity. Frequency of electrical stimulation is modulated from 1 Hz at steady state to 0.5–3 Hz in random increments (at 37 °C). Trabecula contraction is allowed to stabilize at each frequency. In non-failing human myocardial trabeculae, contraction stress should increase with increased stimulation frequency [20]. A negative stress–frequency relationship is a hallmark of failing myocardium [21].
   (d) *Post-pause potentiation:* Surrogate for the balance between sarcoplasmic reticulum (SR) Ca^{2+} uptake, passive SR Ca^{2+} leak, and Ca^{2+} extrusion at rest [6, 15, 22, 23]. Achieved by switching off the electrical stimulation for uniform periods of 2–60 s before resuming at the same stimulation frequency. The stress amplitude of the first post-pause contraction is compared to the last pre-pause contraction. In non-diseased human atrial myocardium, the post-pause contraction is typically potentiated (increased) relative to the pre-rest contraction when the rest interval is ≤60 s. Note that post-pause potentiation values can be highly variable between trabeculae and between donors.

(e) *Post-pause recovery:* Subsequent non-steady-state technique/analysis to post-pause potentiation. Provides a functional correlate for cardiomyocyte capacity to restore balance between SR Ca^{2+} loading and extracellular Ca^{2+} extrusion [22]. Typically, the amplitudes of post-pause contractions 2–10 are measured. Data can be analyzed as raw values normalized to the pre-rest steady-state contraction amplitude or as regression plots of consecutive contraction amplitudes. For example, the amplitude of the next contraction $(n + 1)^{th}$ can be plotted on the y-axis and the amplitude of the preceding contraction (n^{th}) on the x-axis. The regression slope should be positive and close to the regression line. A change in slope is indicative of a change in Ca^{2+} homeostasis.

(f) *Rapid-cooling contractures:* Rapid cooling of human atrial trabeculae from 27–37 °C to <5 °C causes cardiomyocyte contracture principally through emptying of SR Ca^{2+} [20]. Amplitude of the contracture is used as an index for SR Ca^{2+} content in intact multicellular preparations such as human atrial trabeculae. To perform, simultaneously switch off external electrical stimulus and rapidly (within 1 s) switch inflow (e.g., via a three-way valve) to ice-cold KHB. After maximal contracture is achieved, switch back to normal temperature KHB flow and resume electrical stimulation. Contractures are fully reversible and reproducible. Hence, the technique can be performed multiple times in the same preparation. It is important to note that rapid-cooling contracture amplitudes decrease naturally in proportion to developed force during an experiment [24].

(g) *K^+ contracture:* Used to assess myofilament Ca^{2+} sensitivity and cross-bridge kinetics [25]. The superfusate is switched from normal KHB to modified high K^+ (121–142 mM KCl) KHB with supraphysiological Ca^{2+} (6 mM $CaCl_2$) to depolarize the trabecula cardiomyocytes, which causes substantial influx of Ca^{2+} and tetanizes the trabecula into a contracture. The modified superfusate is washed-in for 30–60 s depending on the flow rate. Once in contracture, the electric stimulus is switched off and maximal contracture is allowed to develop. Thereafter, normal KHB superfusion is resumed and stimulation is resumed once contracture is abolished.

16. Contraction frequency is useful for identifying periods of unstimulated (i.e., arrhythmic) trabecula contractions.

17. It is becoming increasingly common to calculate human trabecula stress from absolute force by normalizing to the cardiomyocyte cross-sectional area measured from immunohistochemical or immunocytochemical staining of transverse sections of the same human trabecula [14, 26]. Human cardiac tissues, especially those procured during cardiac surgery from individuals with cardiovascular disease of typically older populations, can contain a profound abundance of non-cardiomyocyte tissues. Hence, if the functional capacity of the contractile cells of the trabecula tissue is being tested by the investigator(s), trabecula force normalization to total trabecula cross-sectional area can be a poor index of myocardial function.
18. It is critical that inclusion and/or exclusion criteria for trabecula analyses are created before beginning a project. These should be stated in the research article. A key criterion is the acceptable extent of trabecula functional degradation over time. Typically, studies have used ≥15–20% per hour reductions in active stress as an exclusion criterion [19, 27]. Separate time-control experiments can be highly useful when determining the normal contractility (or other functional outputs) deterioration on a given system. This is especially prudent if investigating a hypothesized negative inotrope.

References

1. Keon WJ, Taichman GC, Mainwood GW (1984) Human atrial trabeculae: an experimental preparation for studying myocardial response to perioperative manipulations. Can J Surg 27:372–377
2. Lin C-I, Chiu T-H, Chiang BN, Cheng K-K (1985) Electromechanical effects of caffeine in isolated human atrial fibres. Cardiovasc Res 19:727–733
3. Bisping E, Tenderich G, Barckhausen P et al (2007) Atrial myocardium is the predominant inotropic target of adrenomedullin in the human heart. Am J Physiol Heart Circ Physiol 293:H3001–H3007
4. Kockskämper J, Khafaga M, Grimm M et al (2008) Angiotensin II and myosin light-chain phosphorylation contribute to the stretch-induced slow force response in human atrial myocardium. Cardiovasc Res 79:642–651
5. Lareau S, Moore R, Mainwood GW et al (1991) An NMR probe to study function and metabolism simultaneously in isolated human cardiac tissue. Magn Reson Med 20:312–318
6. Sossalla S, Kallmeyer B, Wagner S et al (2010) Altered Na^+ currents in atrial fibrillation: effects of ranolazine on arrhythmias and contractility in human atrial myocardium. J Am Coll Cardiol 55:2330–2342
7. Wettwer E, Christ T, Endig S et al (2013) The new antiarrhythmic drug vernakalant: ex vivo study of human atrial tissue from sinus rhythm and chronic atrial fibrillation. Cardiovasc Res 98:145–154
8. Kentish JC, ter Keurs HE, Ricciardi L et al (1986) Comparison between the sarcomere length-force relations of intact and skinned trabeculae from rat right ventricle: influence of calcium concentrations on these relations. Circ Res 58:755–768
9. Jones TL, Kaur S, Kang N et al (2023) Impaired calcium handling mechanisms in atrial trabeculae of diabetic patients. Physiol Rep 11:e15599
10. Mulieri LA, Hasenfuss G, Ittleman F et al (1989) Protection of human left ventricular myocardium from cutting injury with 2, 3-butanedione monoxime. Circ Res 65:1441–1449
11. Pecha S, Geelhoed B, Kempe R et al (2021) No impact of sex and age on beta-adrenoceptor-mediated inotropy in human right atrial trabeculae. Acta Physiol 231:e13564

12. Pecha S, Ismaili D, Geelhoed B et al (2023) Resting membrane potential is less negative in trabeculae from right atrial appendages of women, but action potential duration does not shorten with age. J Mol Cell Cardiol 176:1–10
13. Raman S, Kelley MA, Janssen PM (2006) Effect of muscle dimensions on trabecular contractile performance under physiological conditions. Pflugers Arch 451:625–630
14. Pecha S, Koivumäki J, Geelhoed B et al (2018) Normalization of force to muscle cross-sectional area: a helpful attempt to reduce data scattering in contractility studies? Acta Physiol 224:e13202
15. Lebek S, Plößl A, Baier M et al (2018) The novel CaMKII inhibitor GS-680 reduces diastolic SR ca leak and prevents CaMKII-dependent pro-arrhythmic activity. J Mol Cell Cardiol 118:159–168
16. Torres CA, Varian KD, Canan CH et al (2013) The positive inotropic effect of pyruvate involves an increase in myofilament calcium sensitivity. PLoS One 8:e63608
17. Babakr AA, Fomison-Nurse IC, van Hout I et al (2020) Acute interaction between human epicardial adipose tissue and human atrial myocardium induce arrhythmic susceptibility. Am J Physiol Endocrinol Metab 218:E164–E172
18. Vermeulen JT, Mcguire MA, Opthof T et al (1994) Triggered activity and automaticity in ventricular trabeculae of failing human and rabbit hearts. Cardiovasc Res 28:1547–1554
19. Aitken-Buck HM, Krause J, van Hout I et al (2021) Long-chain acylcarnitine 18:1 acutely increases human atrial myocardial contractility and arrhythmia susceptibility. Am J Physiol Heart Circ Physiol 321:H162–HH74
20. Maier LS, Barckhausen P, Weisser J et al (2000) Ca^{2+} handling in isolated human atrial myocardium. Am J Phsyiol Heart Circ Physiol 27:952–958
21. Pieske B, Maier LS, Bers DM et al (1999) Ca^{2+} handling and sarcoplasmic reticulum Ca^{2+} content in isolated failing and nonfailing human myocardium. Circ Res 85:38–46
22. Ravens U, Gath J, Hussaini MA et al (1997) Mechanical restitution in atrial muscle from human and rat hearts: effects of agents that modify sarcoplasmic reticulum function. Pharmacol Toxicol 81:97–104
23. Aitken-Buck HM, Babakr AA, Fomison-Nurse IC et al (2020) Inotropic and lusitropic, but not arrhythmogenic, effects of adipocytokine resistin on human atrial myocardium. Am Heart Physiol Endocrinol Metab 319:E540–E547
24. Milani-Nejad N, Brunello L, Gyorke S et al (2014) Decrease in sarcoplasmic reticulum calcium content, not myofilament function, contributes to muscle twitch force decline in isolated cardiac trabeculae. J Muscle Res Cell Motil 35:225–234
25. Varian KD, Raman S, Janssen PM (2006) Measurement of myofilament calcium sensitivity at physiological temperature in intact cardiac trabeculae. Am J Physiol Heart Circ Physiol 290: H2092–H2097
26. Munro ML, Shen X, Ward M et al (2018) Highly variable contractile performance correlates with myocyte content in trabeculae from failing human hearts. Sci Rep 8:2957
27. Janssen PM, Zeitz O, Keweloh B et al (2000) Influence of cyclosporine a on contractile function, calcium handling, and energetics in isolated human and rabbit myocardium. Cardiovasc Res 47:99–107

Chapter 7

Measurement of Intracellular Ca^{2+} in Muscle Isolated from Rat and Human Hearts

Amelia S. Power and Marie-Louise Ward

Abstract

Contraction and relaxation within the heart is controlled by the coordinated rise and fall of Ca^{2+} levels within the cytosol of cardiomyocytes. This requires Ca^{2+} to be moved between subcellular and extracellular compartments with each cardiac cycle, since Ca^{2+} is not destroyed or broken down by the excitation–contraction and relaxation cycles. Many cardiac pathologies alter Ca^{2+} homeostasis and can lead to impaired contraction, incomplete relaxation, and arrhythmias. Ca^{2+}-sensitive fluorescent probes enable monitoring of Ca^{2+} cycling and can be used to detect pathological changes that can then be investigated using novel therapeutic strategies in isolated heart cells and tissues. This chapter will describe simultaneous measurements of intracellular Ca^{2+} using the ratiometric indicator fura-2/AM, and contractile force in isolated multicellular muscles (trabeculae) dissected from rat hearts, or from viable samples of human right atrial appendage.

Key words Calcium ion (Ca^{2+}), Excitation, contraction coupling, Cardiac muscle function, Fluorescence, Fura-2, Trabecula

1 Introduction

Muscle was first found to contract in response to electrical stimulation more than 200 years ago by Luigi Galvani [1], and our current understanding of the fundamental properties of the excitable cells originates from experiments performed by Hodgkin and Huxley in the 1950s [2]. The work of Ringer (1883) in the late nineteenth century showed that Ca^{2+} in the extracellular solution bathing heart tissue was required for sustained contractility [3]. The mechanisms underlying cardiac excitation–contraction coupling (ECC) and the role of Ca^{2+} are now well understood, in health [4] and disease states [5–7].

ECC depends critically on the expression of key Ca^{2+} proteins, and their subcellular localization, which is reviewed extensively elsewhere [8]. In brief, following depolarization of the surface sarcolemma and transverse tubules, the voltage-dependent L-type

Dhananjie N. K. Chandrasekera and Rajesh Katare (eds.), *Cardiomyocytes: Methods and Protocols*, Methods in Molecular Biology, vol. 2894, https://doi.org/10.1007/978-1-0716-4342-6_7,

Ca^{2+} channels open causing an influx of Ca^{2+} known as the "Ca^{2+} current." The Ca^{2+} current then triggers opening of the ryanodine receptors (RyR2) on the junctional sarcoplasmic reticulum (SR) in a process termed Ca^{2+}-induced Ca^{2+} release [9]. The SR Ca^{2+}-release rapidly results in a tenfold increase in the cytosolic Ca^{2+} concentration, initiating the upstroke of the "Ca^{2+} transient." Ca^{2+} then diffuses to the contractile proteins, activating cross-bridge cycling and force production. Relaxation occurs when the cytosolic Ca^{2+} concentration returns again to resting levels. For this to happen, Ca^{2+} is mainly re-sequestered back into the SR by the SR Ca^{2+} ATPase (SERCA), with a smaller amount transported back out of the cell via the Na^+/Ca^{2+} exchanger (NCX). During steady-state conditions, the amount of Ca^{2+} transported out of the myocytes during diastole by NCX must be equal to the amount entering during the Ca^{2+} current [8]. However, the relative contributions of key proteins to Ca^{2+} cycling can be altered to match the changing metabolic demands experienced in our daily lives [10].

It is now widely established that the coordinated cycling of intracellular Ca^{2+}, initiated by the cardiomyocyte action potential, on a beat-to-beat basis is vital to the proper function of the heart. Disruption of Ca^{2+} homeostasis can lead to weaker contractions (heart failure with reduced ejection fraction), incomplete relaxation (heart failure with preserved ejection fraction), and uncoordinated contraction events (arrhythmias) [11, 12]. Considerable research is now focused on restoring Ca^{2+} handling in heart failure by both genetic and pharmacological interventions [13].

The first optical measurements of Ca^{2+} transients were made by microinjecting the Ca^{2+}-sensitive bioluminescent protein aequorin into frog atrial trabeculae [14]. Allen and Blinks (1978) demonstrated that increased trabeculae tension with inotropic interventions was accompanied by increased Ca^{2+} transient amplitude [14]. It is now understood that the size and time course of the Ca^{2+} transient are critical to contractile function [15, 16] and that the dynamic balance of Ca^{2+} cycling can be altered by many factors, such as stimulation frequency (heart rate) [14, 17], catecholamines [14, 18] sarcomere length [19], and many pathological conditions [20, 21].

1.1 Fura-2

Although aequorin measurements of intracellular Ca^{2+} in cardiac muscle preparations advanced our understanding of cardiomyocyte function, there were many disadvantages in its use. The development of Ca^{2+}-sensitive fluorescent indicators by Tsien [22] and co-workers [23] in the 1980s revolutionized our ability to monitor intracellular Ca^{2+} fluctuations in biological preparations for longer periods of time. Fura-2 is a commonly used Ca^{2+}-sensitive fluorophore for measurements of intracellular Ca^{2+} in cardiac muscle preparations. It has an in vitro K_d of ~371 nM [24], making it the most sensitive within the normal range of cytosolic Ca^{2+} fluxes

(~10 nM to ~1 μM) in cardiomyocytes [25]. There is a spectral shift in peak emitted fluorescence for fura-2, dependent on whether Ca^{2+} is bound (peak at 340 nm) or not (peak at 380 nm), making it suitable for ratiometric measurements. The isosbestic point for fura-2 excitation is 360 nm, where emitted fluorescence is independent of [Ca^{2+}], enabling it to be used as a reference for the amount of indicator in the cytosol following loading when compared to the autofluorescence value at 360 nm. Therefore, the ratio of emitted fluorescence (~510 nm) from 340 nm excitation over 380 nm excitation reports the $[Ca^{2+}]_i$ which is independent of fura-2-concentration within the cells. Use of a ratiometric indicator has many advantages, such as elimination of variations due to uneven dye concentration, leakage of dye with time, photobleaching, changes in cell volume, and movement artifacts.

There are two methods commonly used to load fura-2 into the cytosol of trabeculae cardiomyocytes: (1) iontophoretic loading of the fura-2 K^+ salt [26] or (2) use of the membrane permeable acetoxy-methyl (AM) form of fura-2 [27]. This chapter will describe the second method where fura-2/AM is added to the trabeculae superfusate since in our hands, it is less damaging to the muscles. During loading, fura-2/AM passively diffuses into the cardiomyocytes where it is de-esterified by cytosolic esterases to the impermeable Ca^{2+}-sensitive form of fura-2 [28]. By slowly loading trabeculae at room temperature, the risk of dye entering the subcellular compartments is minimized.

1.2 Cardiac Trabeculae

Trabeculae are free-running, cylindrical (or elliptical) multicellular muscles suitable for simultaneous measurements of intracellular Ca^{2+} and force. Trabeculae are continuously superfused with oxygenated buffer solutions and should therefore have radii that are less than ~100 μm to prevent cardiomyocytes at the center from becoming anoxic [29]. Cardiomyocytes are aligned along the length of trabeculae (Fig. 1F), making them suitable for isometric force measurements [30]. This chapter will detail the methods of fura-2 loading and fluorescence measurements obtained from both rat and human trabeculae.

2 Materials

2.1 Microdissection of Trabeculae

1. A double-walled, custom-made dissection bath with a SYLGARD base to the inner chamber and an inflow cannula of 2.5 mm diameter (for adult rat heart aorta; Fig. 1A) connected via Tygon® tubing and MiniPuls Gilson pump to the buffer reservoir. The inner chamber of the dissection bath has a 1 cm notch in the top edge to allow overflow of buffer solution which drains to waste via the outer chamber. The 1 L reservoir containing dissection buffer is constantly bubbled with

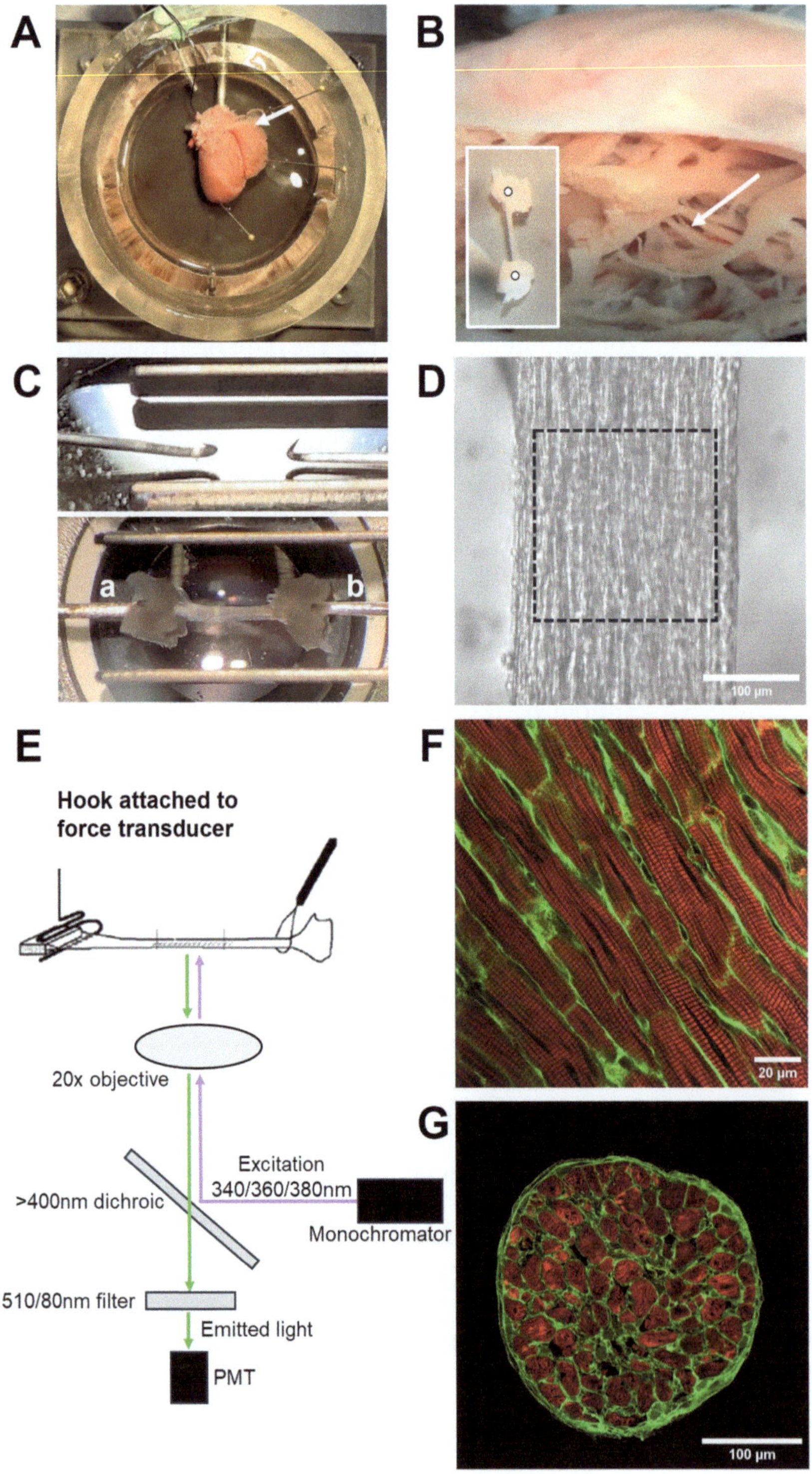

Fig. 1 Trabeculae dissection and imaging set up. (**A**) Shows the dissection bath with a rat heart aorta cannulated and RV-free wall opened to reveal the location (white arrow) where trabeculae suitable for microdissection are typically found. (**B**) Shows the endocardial surface of a human right atrial appendage. A

carbogen gas (5% CO_2, 95% O_2) using a glass tube with a gas dispersion tip, with buffer continuously supplied to the rat heart aorta via the cannula, or by directly flooding the chamber to keep tissues well oxygenated during dissection.

2. Dissection microscope with 7–30× magnification (SMZ-1B, Nikon, Japan) and a double-headed cold light with distensible arms to illuminate the endocardial surface (LG-PS2, Olympus, Japan).
3. Stainless steel insect pins (0.5 and 0.25 mm diameter).
4. 2× Dumont #5 forceps (11252-30, Fine Science Tools, Germany) and Vannas spring scissors with 2.5 and 4 mm cutting edge (15000-08 and 15018-10, Fine Science Tools). For cannulation of the rat heart aorta, 2× Taylor forceps and size 3/0 silk suture are required (11011-17 and 18020-30, Fine Science Tools).
5. 0.1 mL plastic spoon (F36721-0010, SP Bel-Art, USA) for transferring the dissected trabeculae to the muscle chamber on the inverted microscope stage.

2.2 Muscle Chamber and Fluorescence System

1. Small intact fiber test apparatus (Model 801C, Aurora Scientific, Canada) with a thermometer/TEC controller (Model 826A, Aurora Scientific) sitting on an inverted microscope (Eclipse TE2000-U, Nikon, Japan) stage above an S fluor 20×/0.75 objective (Nikon). A separate dissection microscope (SMZ-1B, Nikon) is mounted above the inverted microscope to help position the preparations. The entire apparatus must be housed in a space which can be shielded from ambient light.
2. Isometric force measurements are made using an AE801 sensor with custom-made hook with ~2 cm extension glued to the silicon beam. The hook is made from a 0.25 mm stainless steel dissection pin and mounted to the micromanipulator on the left-hand side of the small intact fiber test apparatus (Fig. 1C, a). A similar hook is glued to a beam mounted onto the right-hand micromanipulator (Fig. 1C, b). Other forms of mounting

Fig. 1 (continued) suitable free-running trabecula is indicated by the white arrow, with a dissected trabecula (inset) showing tissue blocks at each end with needle punctures (open circles) for mounting to the bath hooks. (**C**) Bath hooks before and after mounting a trabecula are shown, with (**a**) indicating hook extending from the force transducer, and (**b**) fixed to a micromanipulator, all sitting above a 20× objective. (**D**) An image from a mounted trabecula with the central portion (dotted square) selected by adjusting the apertures to create a field of view for collecting emitted fluorescence. (**E**) Shows a schematic diagram of the light paths of excitation and emitted fura-2 fluorescence. (**F**) A confocal image obtained from a 10 μm longitudinal section of a rat RV trabecula fixed and labeled post-experimentation to show myofilaments (red, phalloidin) and extracellular matrix (green, wheat germ agglutinin). (**G**) A confocal image of a 10 μm transverse section through a rat RV trabecula, prepared as in (**F**) trabeculae can also be used; we find the simple hooks shown in Fig. 1C are suitable for mounting human trabeculae. The hook shown in Fig. 1E is more suitable for rat trabeculae where the tissue blocks are generally less fibrotic, and the other end of the trabecula is held with a snare around the valve tissue which is made with a blunted 30 G needle threaded with monofilament suture.

3. An Optoscan monochromator (Cairn Research, Faversham, UK) equipped with a light source (75 W xenon arc lamp) and power supply, monochromator, Optoscan control unit, and photomultiplier tube (PMT) mounted to the left-hand port of the microscope. The xenon arc lamp provides a stable white light that is passed through the monochromator and separated into specific excitation bandwidths. For fura-2, the monochromator is programmed to cycle through excitation wavelengths of 340, 360, and 380 nm (with 10 nm bandwidth) each for a duration of 5 ms. Emitted light above 400 nm is passed through a dichroic (400DCLP, Chroma Technology, USA) and then collected by the PMT fitted with a 510/80 nm filter (D510/80 M, Chroma Technology) (Fig. 1E).
4. Trabeculae are electrically stimulated using a Radnoti RAD-STIM multichannel stimulator (ADInstruments, New Zealand) connected to the platinum plate electrodes of the small intact fiber test apparatus and along the length of the bath parallel to the mounting hooks (Fig. 1C).
5. A MiniPuls Gilson pump with inflow and outflow tubing connected to the small intact fiber test apparatus set to deliver a flow at a rate of 3 mL/min and total dead space of 6 mL including the pump tubing and muscle bath (*see* **Note 1**).
6. A PowerLab data acquisition system (8/35, ADInstruments) is used to obtain isometric force, emitted fluorescence at three different excitation wavelengths (three channels), stimulus voltage, and ratio (340/380) data, recorded using LabChart 8 software (ADInstruments).

2.3 Preparation of Buffers and Reagents

All solutions are prepared with distilled H_2O and, unless otherwise stated, they are made in advance and stored at room temperature.

1. Krebs–Henseleit buffer (KHB): 118.5 mM NaCl, 4.5 mM KCl, 156 mM NaH_2PO_4, 1 $MgCl_2$, 25 mM $NaHCO_3$, 11 mM D(+)glucose (*see* **Note 2**).
2. Collection, dissection, and mounting buffer: 25 mM 2,3-butanedione monoxime (BDM) in KHB buffer. On the day of the experiment, dissolve 2.252 g BDM and 1.982 g glucose in 1 L of KHB and place on stir plate to dissolve.

(a) *Human tissue collection*: Add 100 mL to a Schutt bottle and bubble with carbogen before addition of 0.25 mM $CaCl_2$ (25 μL of 1 M $CaCl_2$ stock). Continuously bubble using an anesthetic bag containing carbogen, and transport on ice to the surgical theatre to collect a freshly excised piece of right atrial appendage tissue from a consenting patient undergoing coronary artery bypass graft surgery.

(b) *Rat heart collection*: Add 50 mL of buffer to a small metal bowl and allow to chill in the freezer prior to collecting a freshly excised rat heart.

(c) *Dissection bath*: Add 800 mL of buffer to the dissection reservoir and saturate with carbogen before the addition of 0.25 mM $CaCl_2$ (200 μL of 1 M $CaCl_2$ stock). Prime inflow tubing to the dissection bath so there are no air bubbles.

(d) *Muscle chamber for mounting*: Add 100 mL to a cylinder and bubble with carbogen before the addition of 0.5 mM $CaCl_2$ (50 μL of 1 M $CaCl_2$ stock). Circulate the bubbled solution through the muscle bath at a flow rate of 3 mL/min.

3. Prepare an additional 100 mL cylinder of regular KHB (without BDM) and bubble with carbogen before the addition of 0.5 mM $CaCl_2$ (50 μL of 1 M $CaCl_2$ stock) (*see* **Note 3**).
4. 10 μM fura-2 loading solution: Remove 4 mL from the solution prepared in the previous step and add to a 50 mL Falcon tube. Bring two 50 μg vials of fura-2/AM to room temperature and add 20 μL of anhydrous DMSO to each vial, pipette up and down to mix, and then add 50 μL of PowerLoad™ concentrate (100×) to each vial and mix. Transfer the contents of each vial to the Falcon tube. Finally, add 1 μL of antifoam Y-30 emulsion to the loading solution and keep bubbled with carbogen (*see* **Note 4**).
5. R_{min} calibration solution: 118 mM NaCl, 6 mM KCl, 1.18 mM $MgSO_4$, 1.18 mM KH_2PO_4, 24.8 mM $NaHCO_3$, 10 mM caffeine, 10 mM BDM, 10 mM ethylene glycol-bis(-β-aminoethyl)-N,N,N′,N′-tetraacetic acid, 10 mM glucose, 1 mM ouabain, 0.1 mM 2,5-di(tert-butyl)-1,4-benzohydoquinone (TBQ), 1 mM probenecid. Bubbled with carbogen.
6. R_{max} calibration solution: 120 mM LiCl, 1.18 mM $MgSO_4$, 1.18 mM KH_2PO_4, 20 mM $NaHCO_3$, 4.82 mM $KHCO_3$, 10 mM caffeine, 10 mM BDM, 10 mM glucose, 1 mM ouabain, 0.1 mM TBQ, 0.01 mM Br-A23187, 2 mM $CaCl_2$, 1 mM probenecid. Bubbled with carbogen.

3 Methods

3.1 Trabeculae Dissection and Mounting

For rat right ventricular trabeculae dissection, follow ***steps 1–5****:*

1. Immediately following euthanasia, excise the rat heart and place in the chilled collection buffer to rinse blood and dissect off any tissue from around the aorta.
2. Transfer heart to the dissection bath, cannulate aorta, and secure with suture before starting pump to begin perfusion at a flow rate of 4 mL/min.
3. Align the heart with the right ventricle (RV) on the right side of the dissection bath and fix in place with a pin though the apex of the heart.
4. Under a dissection microscope, cut across the right atria to identify the tricuspid valve opening into the RV. Insert the scissors through the valve into the RV, parallel and close to the septum at the edge of the RV free wall and cut toward the apex, and then peel back and pin the RV-free wall to secure it to the SYLGARD base of the dissection dish (Fig. 1A).
5. Identify a suitable, unbranched, free-running trabecula (<200 μm diameter), usually running between the AV valve and the free wall. Using micro-scissors and sharp forceps, cut blocks of tissue containing the free wall and valve end of the trabecula while being careful not to touch the body of the trabecula (Fig. 1B, inset).

For human right atrial appendage trabeculae dissection, follow ***steps*** *6–8:*

6. Immediately following dissection of the right atrial appendage in surgery, transfer the tissue to the collection buffer and rapidly transport to the laboratory (~7 min) while continuously bubbling with carbogen and keeping chilled on ice.
7. Transfer tissue piece to the dissection bath and secure to the SYLGARD base with three to four insect pins.
8. Identify suitable unbranched trabeculae (Fig. 1B, white arrow). Using micro-scissors and sharp forceps, cut blocks of tissue each end of the trabecula while being careful not to touch the body of the trabecula.

Continue for both rat and human trabeculae for using simple hooks as in Fig. 1C*:*

9. Create holes in tissue blocks using the 0.5 mm insect pin (Fig. 1B, insert, white circles).

10. Handling only the blocks of tissue with fine tipped forceps, float the trabecula into a plastic spoon and transfer to the muscle bath on the stage of an inverted microscope with the circulation pump paused.
11. Gently mount the block ends between the two pin hooks so that the trabecula is not stretched (Fig. 1C) and then restart the circulation and start recording in LabChart.
12. Allow muscle to recover for 10 min while continuously superfusing with mounting buffer. During this time, bring the muscle into focus on the inverted microscope and visualize using the microscope camera (Fig. 1D).
13. Switch the circulating superfusate to regular 100 mL KHB with 0.5 mM $CaCl_2$ and monitor baseline force.
14. Once the force has stabilized (~5 min), increase the $CaCl_2$ concentration to 1 mM by pipetting 50 μL of 1 M stock $CaCl_2$ and monitor baseline force.
15. Once the force has stabilized again, begin continuous stimulation of the trabecula at 0.2 Hz (biphasic, 5 ms duration, constant voltage 1.2× stimulation threshold) (*see* **Note 5**).
16. Wait for the contraction amplitude to stabilize and then incrementally increase the length of the trabeculae by moving the pin hook away from the force transducer hook using the right-hand side micromanipulator. Continue to monitor contraction amplitude increasing the trabecula length until there is no further increase in amplitude, and the optimal length (L_o) of the muscle is established.
17. Measure the trabecula diameter (d) using a calibrated graticule and the CCD camera display (Fig. 1D), and calculate the cross-sectional area of the muscle (cylindrical trabeculae, $A = \pi\left(\frac{d}{2}\right)^2$).
18. For an elliptical trabecula, estimate the diameter of the short (a) and wide (b) diameters of the muscle to calculate the cross-sectional area (elliptical trabeculae, $A = \pi\left(\frac{a}{2}\right)\left(\frac{b}{2}\right)$).
19. Add a channel in LabChart data acquisition software to output the stress (mN mm^{-2}) produced by the muscle, using the arithmetic function in channel settings (force/A).

3.2 Fura-2 Loading and Intracellular Ca^{2+} Measurements

1. Using a camera, create a field of view with the aperture adjustments on the emitted light path that encompasses the central portion of the trabecula without capturing the tissue edges (Fig. 1D, dotted square).
2. Switch on the lamp power supply and Optoscan controller rack to warm up 30 min before measurements are collected.

3. Set up the monochromator to sequentially excite the muscle at 340, 360, and 380 nm wavelengths, as outlined in the "Materials" section.
4. Run the wavelength program in continuous cycle mode and switch on the PMT at 700 V to measure tissue autofluorescence for each excitation wavelength (*see* **Note 6**).
5. Begin fura-2 loading by pausing the superfusate pump and switching the inflow and outflow pump tubing to the Falcon tube containing the fura-2 loading solution. The total volume of the loading solution added to the "dead space" of the muscle chamber and tubing should be 10 mL to obtain a final fura-2/AM concentration of 10 μM.
6. Restart the pump; all emitted fluorescence levels should increase as the fura-2 loading solution mixes with the bath superfusate flowing through the muscle chamber within minutes.
7. Continue circulating the loading solution for 2 h checking the fluorescence every 30 min. Successful loading is indicated by a reduction in the 380 nm fluorescence levels.
8. Wash out the loading solution with fresh buffer solution after 2 h of loading; a measure of the loading success can be obtained by comparing the emitted fluorescence at 360 nm excitation post loading to the 360 nm autofluorescence measurement (assuming no changes have been made to PMT voltage or "window" size in the meantime). We find an increase in emitted fluorescence at 360 nm of five times is ideal (*see* **Note 7**).
9. Following the washout period, slacken the muscle and repeat **step 16** from Subheading 3.1 to confirm the muscle is held at L_o.
10. While recording the fluorescence, recheck the microscope focus for optimal fluorescence measurement, considering that for multicellular trabeculae, the emitted fluorescence will come from cardiomyocytes within the trabecula rather than from the surface endothelial cells.
11. Trabeculae can now undergo specific experimental protocols to test the effects of pharmacological agents, or stimulation protocols on intracellular Ca^{2+} handing and contractility. To limit exposure of the muscle to UV light, it is recommended that the wavelength program is switched off between interventions. An example of raw data collected from a fura-2-loaded rat RV trabecula stimulated at 1 Hz is shown in Fig. 2 (*see* **Note 8**).

Optional calibration:

12. Following the experimental protocols, switch off stimulation and switch the superperfusate solution to the R_{min} calibration

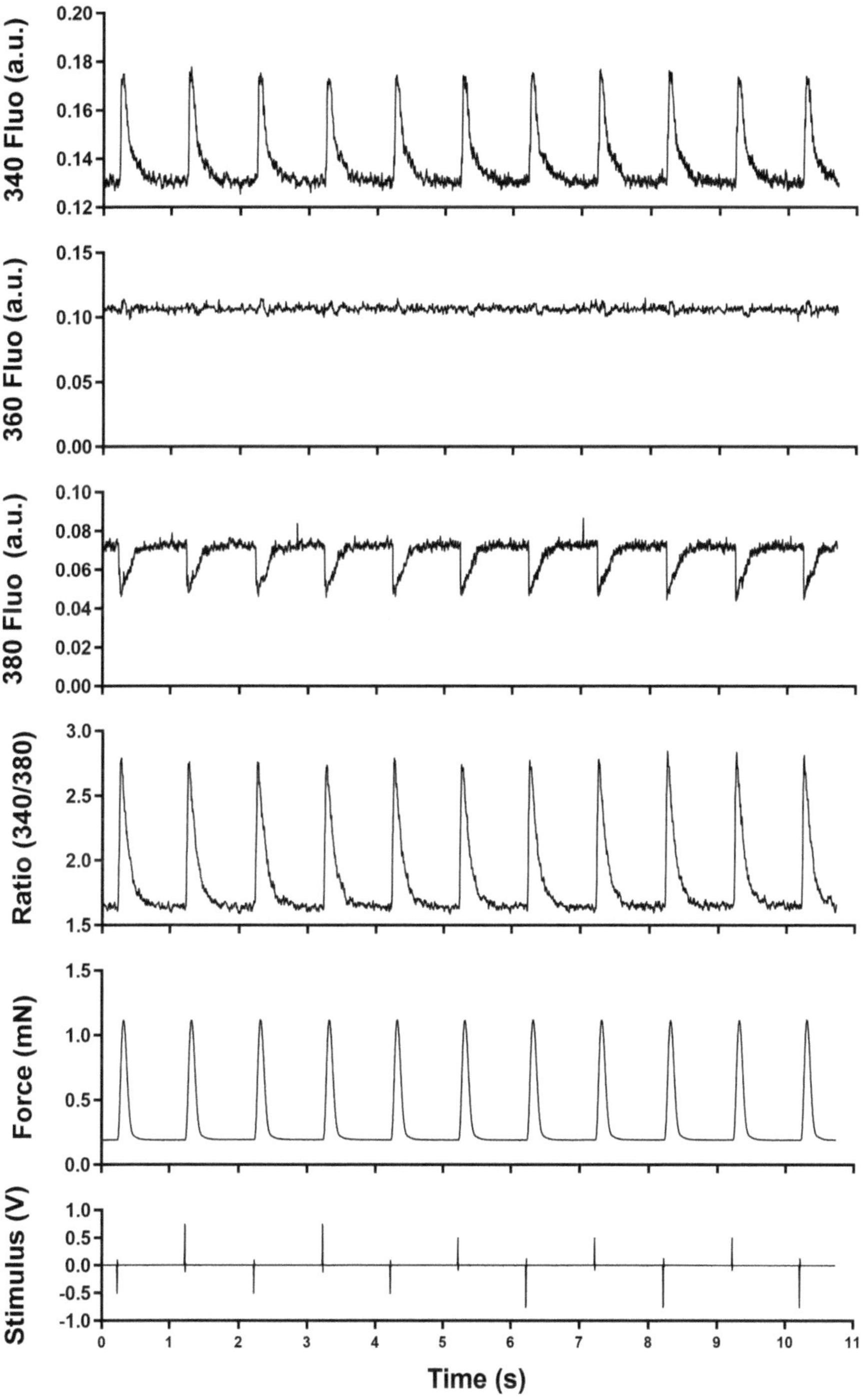

Fig. 2 Example of continuous steady-state measurements made from rat right ventricular trabecula. This figure shows a recording of five variables obtained from a cardiac trabecula producing steady-state Ca^{2+} transients and twitch force at 1 Hz stimulation frequency. The top three traces show emitted fluorescence when excited at wavelengths of 340, 360, and 380 nm, respectively. Note that the 360 nm excitation wavelength is Ca^{2+} independent. The fourth trace shows the resultant 340/380 ratio. The fifth trace shows isometric force at optimal length. Finally, the sixth trace shows alternating stimulus voltage which is used to align the twitches for averaging and calculating time-to-peak Ca^{2+} and force in the peak analysis

solution and allow to equilibrate checking fluorescence values every 10 min until a plateau is reached (~30 min). This solution is designed to deplete the SR and intracellular Ca^{2+} to its minimum concentration.

13. Once the minimum fluorescence ratio is reached, switch the superperfusate to the R_{max} calibration solution and allow to equilibrate (~5 min) while recording the fluorescence.

3.3 Data Analysis

1. Use the peak analysis plugin in LabChart to determine peak parameters from the stress and fura-2 ratio channels.
2. Highlight ~10 (or more/less) sequential responses in the stress or fura-2 ratio channel during steady-state conditions of an experimental protocol and select the Peak Analysis Settings button.
3. Under setup, use the following settings:
   (a) Analysis type: General Unstimulated.
   (b) Source: Stress or fura-2 ratio.
   (c) Selection option chosen.
   (d) Peak detection settings Preset: General—Sine shape.
   (e) Detection adjustment: 2 S.D. (can be modified to change sensitivity).
4. Click on the table view and export parameters for offline analysis:
   (a) Commonly reported Ca^{2+} transient parameters (Fig. 3a, 340/380) that provide information about Ca^{2+} handling within the tissue include:
      (i) Time from stimulus to peak Ca^{2+}.
      (ii) Resting (diastolic) Ca^{2+} level.
      (iii) Peak (systolic) Ca^{2+}.
      (iv) Ca^{2+} transient amplitude.
      (v) Tau of Ca^{2+} transient decay.
   (b) Complimentary parameters from the twitch stress (Fig. 3b, mN mm^{-2}) include:
      (i) Time from stimulus to peak stress.
      (ii) Diastolic stress.
      (iii) Systolic stress.
      (iv) Active stress.
      (v) Time from peak to 50% relaxation.

3.4 Calculating Intracellular-Free Ca^{2+} Concentration

1. Use the modified Grynkiewicz equation (Eq. 1) to convert fura-2 340/380 ratio measurements from arbitrary units (a.u.) to intracellular Ca^{2+} concentration [27, 28].

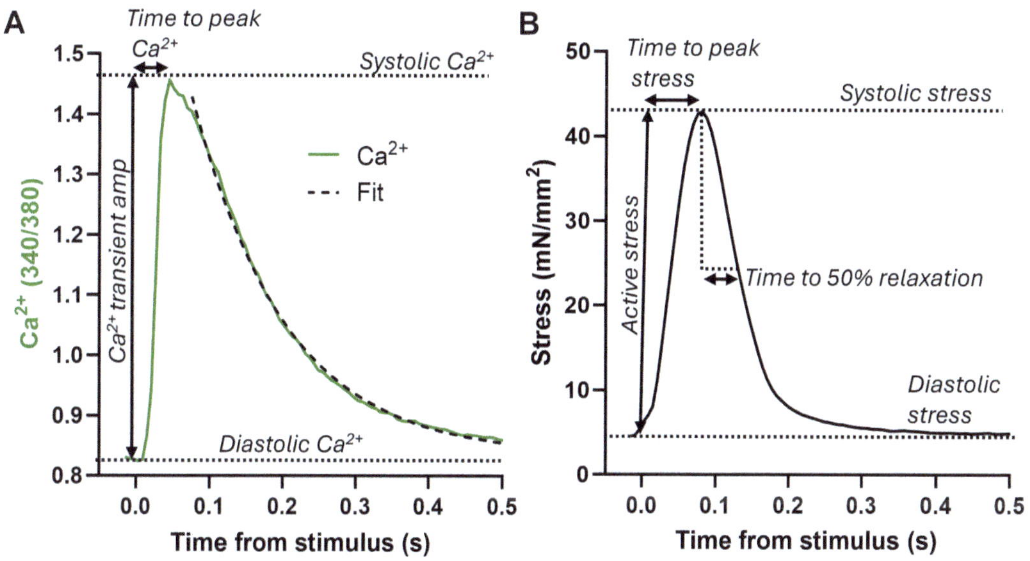

Fig. 3 Force and Ca^{2+} data analysis parameters. Averaged Ca^{2+} transient (**a**) and twitch force normalized to trabecula cross-sectional area (**b**, stress) from ten steady-state responses obtained from a rat RV trabecula stimulated at 1 Hz (time 0 s) at 37 °C. Each average response shows typical parameters obtained for analysis of Ca^{2+} handling and contractile characteristics. The dotted black line in (**a**) is an exponential fitted to the Ca^{2+} transient, used to determine the time constant of Ca^{2+} decay

2. Determine maximum and minimum 340/380 ratio values from trabecula sequentially exposing to R_{min} and R_{max} solutions (Fig. 4a):

$$\left[\mathrm{Ca}^{2+}\right]i = K_d\beta\frac{R - R_{min}}{R_{max} - R} \tag{1}$$

   (a) R is the observed 340/380 ratio.
   (b) R_{min} is the 340/380 ratio following equilibrium with the R_{min} solution.
   (c) R_{max} is the 340/380 ratio following equilibrium with the R_{max} solution.
   (d) K_d is the in vitro dissociation constant of fura-2, determined in cardiomyocytes (0.371 μM) [24].
   (e) β is described below.

3. To account for the loss of indicator during the R_{min} and R_{max} equilibration period [27], calculate β using Eq. 2:

$$\beta = \frac{380R_{min}}{380R_{max}\left(\frac{360R_{min}}{360R_{max}}\right)}. \tag{2}$$

   (a) $380R_{min}$ is the emitted fluorescence when excited at 380 following equilibrium with the R_{min} solution.
   (b) $360R_{min}$ is the emitted fluorescence when excited at 360 following equilibrium with the R_{min} solution.

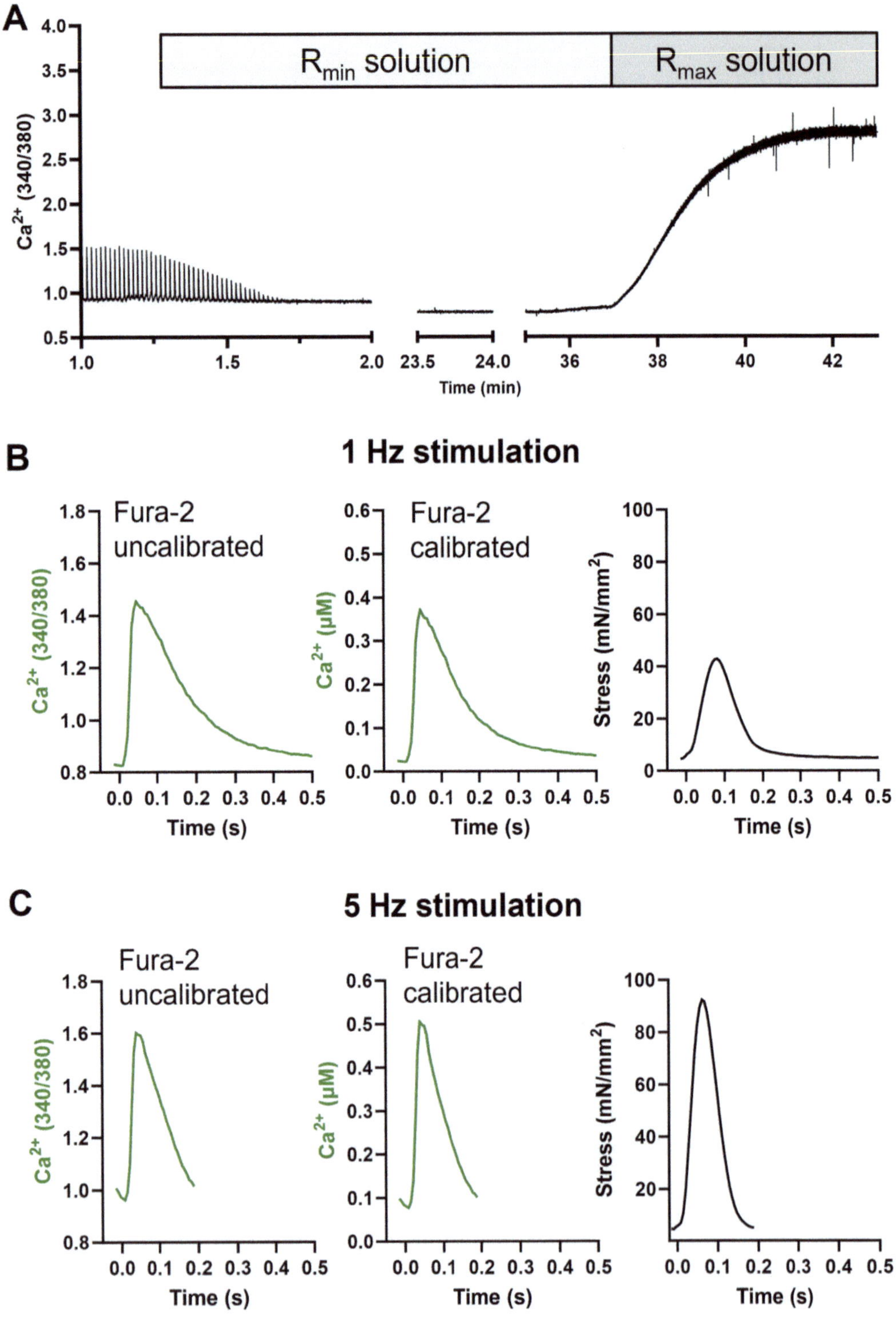

Fig. 4 Fura-2 calibration using R_{min} and R_{max} solutions to determine intracellular Ca^{2+} concentration. (**a**) fura-2 ratio (340/380) recording from a rat RV trabecula before and during exposure to R_{min} and R_{max} solutions that deplete intracellular Ca^{2+} and induce saturating intracellular Ca^{2+}, concentrations, respectively, for calibration of the fura-2 ratio using a modified Grynkiewicz equation. (**b, c**) examples of the fura-2 ratio before and after calibration with simultaneous measurement of stress from the trabecula stimulated at 1 Hz (**b**) and 5 Hz (**c**)

(c) $380R_{max}$ is the emitted fluorescence when excited at 380 following equilibrium with the R_{max} solution.

(d) $360R_{max}$ is the emitted fluorescence when excited at 360 following equilibrium with the R_{max} solution.

3.5 Exemplary Data

1. Examples of the calibrated and uncalibrated ratio data are shown for comparison in a rat trabecula stimulated at 1 and 5 Hz (Fig. 4b, c). Notably, with an increase in stimulation frequency, there is an increase in both systolic and diastolic Ca^{2+} indicating a greater release of Ca^{2+} from the SR (Table 1). The time to peak Ca^{2+} is shorter indicating faster release of Ca^{2+} at 5 Hz, and the tau of Ca^{2+} decay is also shorter indicating faster uptake of Ca^{2+} back into the SR. The changes in the Ca^{2+} transient translate to a twofold increase in active stress at 5 Hz, as well as faster development of stress and accelerated relaxation of the trabecula to accommodate the increased frequency of contraction typical of a healthy RV trabecula [6].
2. Examples of averaged force and uncalibrated Ca^{2+} from a human right atrial appendage trabeculae are shown in Fig. 5 when stimulated at 1 Hz and treated with the experimental drug

Table 1
Representative Ca^{2+} and force parameters measured from a rat trabecula under different stimulation frequencies with 1.5 mM extracellular Ca^{2+} at 37 °C

	Rat	
Ca^{2+} parameters	**1 Hz**	**5 Hz**
Systolic Ca^{2+} (340/380) (a.u.)	1.456	1.602
Diastolic Ca^{2+} (340/380) (a.u.)	0.824	0.962
Ca^{2+} transient amplitude (Δ340/380) (a.u.)	0.631	0.640
Systolic Ca^{2+} (μM)	0.372	0.505
Diastolic Ca^{2+} (μM)	0.022	0.078
Ca^{2+} transient amplitude (μM)	0.350	0.427
Time-to-peak Ca^{2+} (s)	0.045	0.033
Tau of Ca^{2+} decay (s)	0.110	0.091
Force parameters		
Systolic stress (mN mm^{-2})	42.9	92.3
Diastolic stress (mN mm^{-2})	4.5	5.6
Active stress (ΔmN mm^{-2})	38.4	86.7
Time to peak stress (s)	0.081	0.063
Time to 50% relaxation (s)	0.048	0.036

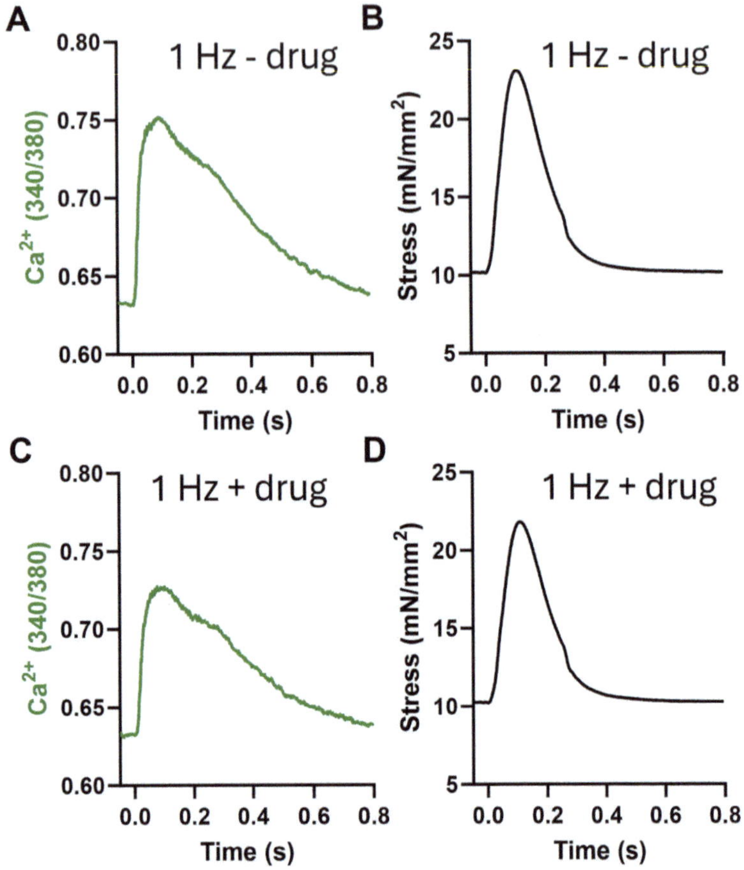

Fig. 5 Representative Ca^{2+} transients and twitch stress from a human right atrial appendage trabecula before and during exposure to drug. Averaged Ca^{2+} transient and twitch stress from a human trabecula, before (**a**, **b**) and during exposure to the mitochondrial Na^{+}/Ca^{+} exchanger inhibitor (**c**, **d**; 5 μM CGP-37157). Trabeculae were stimulated at 1 Hz, with 1.5 mM extracellular Ca^{2+}, at 37 °C

CGP-37157 (5 μM, Sigma-Aldrich), a selective inhibitor of the mitochondrial Na^{+}/Ca^{2+} exchanger. The human atrial Ca^{2+} transients are markedly slower in comparison to the rat trabeculae, and the measured Ca^{2+} and stress parameters are summarized in Table 2.

4 Notes

1. It is important to use tubing with low O_2 permeability between the oxygenated KHB cylinder and the muscle chamber (we use Tygon® R3603, internal diameter 1 mm, external diameter 4 mm). To maintain a constant level of buffer in the muscle chamber, we use outflow tubing of slightly larger internal diameter connected to a stainless tube with a beveled tip (18 G

Table 2
Representative Ca^{2+} and force parameters calculated from a human right atrial trabecula before and during drug exposure (5 μM CGP-37157) with 1.5 mM extracellular Ca^{2+} at 37 °C

	Human	
Ca^{2+} parameters	**1 Hz − drug**	**1 Hz + drug**
Systolic Ca^{2+} (340/380) (a.u.)	0.752	0.727
Diastolic Ca^{2+} (340/380) (a.u.)	0.631	0.631
Ca^{2+} transient amplitude (Δ340/380) (a.u.)	0.120	0.096
Time to peak Ca^{2+} (s)	0.091	0.076
Tau of Ca^{2+} decay (s)	0.532	0.565
Force parameters		
Systolic stress (mN mm^{-2})	23.1	21.8
Diastolic stress (mN mm^{-2})	10.2	10.2
Active stress (ΔmN mm^{-2})	13.0	11.6
Time-to-peak stress (s)	0.105	0.109
Time to 50% relaxation (s)	0.102	0.101

hypodermic needle) for the outflow. The tip of the bevel then sits on the meniscus of the buffer such that air and buffer are pumped back to the reservoir.

2. Ca^{2+} and glucose-free KHB can be made in large volumes (10 L) and stored at room temperature until the day of experimentation. Addition of glucose can be made on the day of experimentation, and Ca^{2+} added to bicarbonate-buffered solutions once they have been equilibrated with carbogen (95% O_2 and 5% CO_2) to maintain a pH of 7.4. Alternatively, HEPES-based Tyrode's buffer can also be used where pH is set to 7.4 with NaOH and the solution is bubbled with 100% O_2.
3. For human atrial trabeculae, supplementation of the regular KHB with 5 mM sodium pyruvate improves the contractile response (trabeculae producing more than 0.5 mN mm^{-2} at 1 Hz, $[Ca^{2+}]_o$ 1.5 mM, 37 °C).
4. Prewarming of the DMSO helps dissolve the fura-2 and to maximize the transfer of fura-2 into the loading solution. PowerLoad can cause foaming of the loading solution during bubbling. This is prevented by adding anti-foam, which should be kept to the minimum volume to prevent excessive foaming. The 4 mL volume of loading solution can be adjusted to accommodate the dead space of the tubing and muscle bath (total

volume should be 10 mL); however, the volume in the Falcon tube should not be less than 3.5 mL to maintain oxygenation of the superfusate.

5. For human trabeculae, the time for stabilization is typically longer (10–15 min), and the temperature controller should be switched on to 37 °C before stimulating the trabeculae. The stimulus voltage required will vary with trabeculae diameter and stimulus duration. We also find human trabeculae typically require a higher stimulus voltage (6–12 V) compared to rat trabeculae (1–4 V) using the Radnoti RADSTIM stimulator.
6. The PMT voltage should be operated within the recommended voltage range and will need to be determined for individual setups depending on the fluorescence values obtained with fura-2 loading. If the signal is saturated (typically occurs in the 380 nm channel as fura-2 produces the most emitted light when excited at 380 nm), then either the "window" size or the PMT voltage can be decreased.
7. The muscle loading should be performed at room temperature to minimize compartmentalization of fura-2 into the SR and mitochondria. For human trabeculae, decreasing the bath temperature to room temperature causes a drop in twitch force during the loading; however, this should recover following washout out of the loading solution when the superfusate is returned to 37 °C.
8. When experiments are performed at 37 °C, the superfusate buffer solutions should be supplemented with 1 mM water-soluble probenecid to inhibit organic-anion transporters that extrude fura-2 from the cytosol. Although the use of ratiometric indicators overcomes changes in the intracellular fluorophore concentration, significant loss of fura-2 signal occurs after 10–15 min at 37 °C unless probenecid is used.

References

1. Piccolino M (1998) Animal electricity and the birth of electrophysiology: the legacy of Luigi Galvani. Brain Res Bull 46(5):381–407
2. Hodgkin AL, Huxley AF (1952) A quantitative description of membrane current and its application to conduction and excitation in nerve. J Physiol 117(4):500–544
3. Ringer S (1883) A further contribution regarding the influence of the different constituents of the blood on the contraction of the heart. J Physiol 4(1):29–42 23
4. Bers DM (2000) Calcium fluxes involved in control of cardiac myocyte contraction. Circ Res 87(4):275–281
5. Jones TLM, Kaur S, Kang N, Ruygrok PN, Ward ML (2023) Impaired calcium handling mechanisms in atrial trabeculae of diabetic patients. Physiol Rep 11(3):e15599. https://doi.org/10.14814/phy2.15599
6. Power A, Hickey A, Crossman D, Loiselle D, Ward ML (2018) Calcium mishandling impairs contraction in right ventricular hypertrophy prior to overt heart failure. Pflugers Arch - Eur J Physiol 7(470):1115–1126
7. Grimm M, Ling H, Willeford A, Pereira L, Gray CB, Erickson JR, Sarma S, Respress JL, Wehrens XH, Bers DM, Brown JH (2015) CaMKIIdelta mediates beta-adrenergic effects on RyR2 phosphorylation and SR Ca(2+) leak and the pathophysiological response to chronic beta-adrenergic stimulation. J Mol Cell Cardiol

85:282–291. https://doi.org/10.1016/j.yjmcc.2015.06.007

8. Eisner DA, Caldwell JL, Kistamas K, Trafford AW (2017) Calcium and excitation-contraction coupling in the heart. Circ Res 121(2):181–195. https://doi.org/10.1161/CIRCRESAHA.117.310230
9. Fabiato A (1983) Calcium-induced release of calcium from the cardiac sarcoplasmic reticulum. Am J Phys 245(1):C1–C14
10. Ward ML, Crossman DJ, Loiselle DS, Cannell MB (2010) Non-steady-state calcium handling in failing hearts from the spontaneously hypertensive rat. Arch Eur J Physiol 460(6):991–1001. https://doi.org/10.1007/s00424-010-0876-3
11. Kilfoil PJ, Lotteau S, Zhang R, Yue X, Aynaszyan S, Solymani RE, Cingolani E, Marbán E, Goldhaber JI (2020) Distinct features of calcium handling and β-adrenergic sensitivity in heart failure with preserved versus reduced ejection fraction. J Physiol 598(22):5091–5108. https://doi.org/10.1113/JP280425
12. Kistamás K, Veress R, Horváth B, Bányász T, Nánási PP, Eisner DA (2020) Calcium handling defects and cardiac arrhythmia syndromes. Front Pharmacol 11. https://doi.org/10.3389/fphar.2020.00072
13. Wehrens XHT, Marks AR (2004) Novel therapeutic approaches for heart failure by normalizing calcium cycling. Nat Rev Drug Discov 3(7):565–574. https://doi.org/10.1038/nrd1440
14. Allen DG, Blinks JR (1978) Calcium transients in aequorin-injected frog cardiac muscle. Nature 273(5663):509–513
15. Bassani JW, Yuan W, Bers DM (1995) Fractional SR Ca release is regulated by trigger Ca and SR Ca content in cardiac myocytes. Am J Phys 268(5 Pt 1):C1313–C1319
16. Eisner DA, Trafford AW, Diaz ME, Overend CL, O'Neill SC (1998) The control of Ca release from the cardiac sarcoplasmic reticulum: regulation versus autoregulation. Cardiovasc Res 38(3):589–604
17. Layland J, Kentish JC (1999) Positive force- and [Ca2+]i-frequency relationships in rat ventricular trabeculae at physiological frequencies. Am J Phys 276(1 Pt 2):H9–H18
18. Ginsburg KS, Bers DM (2004) Modulation of excitation-contraction coupling by isoproterenol in cardiomyocytes with controlled SR Ca2+ load and Ca2+ current trigger. J Physiol 556 (Pt 2):463–480. https://doi.org/10.1113/jphysiol.2003.055384
19. Ward ML, Williams IA, Chu Y, Cooper PJ, Ju YK, Allen DG (2008) Stretch-activated channels in the heart: contributions to length-dependence and to cardiomyopathy. Prog Biophys Mol Biol 97(2–3):232–249. https://doi.org/10.1016/j.pbiomolbio.2008.02.009
20. Benoist D, Stones R, Drinkhill MJ, Benson AP, Yang Z, Cassan C, Gilbert SH, Saint DA, Cazorla O, Steele DS, Bernus O, White E (2012) Cardiac arrhythmia mechanisms in rats with heart failure induced by pulmonary hypertension. Am J Physiol Heart Circ Physiol 302(11):H2381–H2395. https://doi.org/10.1152/ajpheart.01084.2011
21. Bers DM (2006) Altered cardiac myocyte ca regulation in heart failure. Physiology (Bethesda) 21:380–387. https://doi.org/10.1152/physiol.00019.2006
22. Tsien RY (1980) New calcium indicators and buffers with high selectivity against magnesium and protons: design, synthesis, and properties of prototype structures. Biochemistry 19(11):2396–2404. https://doi.org/10.1021/bi00552a018
23. Minta A, Kao JP, Tsien RY (1989) Fluorescent indicators for cytosolic calcium based on rhodamine and fluorescein chromophores. J Biol Chem 264(14):8171–8178
24. Haworth RA, Redon D (1998) Calibration of intracellular Ca transients of isolated adult heart cells labelled with fura-2 by acetoxymethyl ester loading. Cell Calcium 24(4):263–273
25. Bers D (2001) Excitation-contraction coupling and cardiac contractile force, vol 237. Springer
26. Backx PH, Ter Keurs HE (1993) Fluorescent properties of rat cardiac trabeculae microinjected with fura-2 salt. Am J Phys 264(4 Pt 2):H1098–H1110. https://doi.org/10.1152/ajpheart.1993.264.4.H1098
27. Ward ML, Pope AJ, Loiselle DS, Cannell MB (2003) Reduced contraction strength with increased intracellular [Ca2+] in left ventricular trabeculae from failing rat hearts. J Physiol 546 (Pt 2):537–550
28. Grynkiewicz G, Poenie M, Tsien RY (1985) A new generation of Ca2+ indicators with greatly improved fluorescence properties. J Biol Chem 260(6):3440–3450
29. Schouten VJ, ter Keurs HE (1986) The force-frequency relationship in rat myocardium. The influence of muscle dimensions. Arch Eur J Physiol 407(1):14–17
30. Hanley PJ, Young AA, LeGrice IJ, Edgar SG, Loiselle DS (1999) 3-dimensional configuration of perimysial collagen fibres in rat cardiac muscle at resting and extended sarcomere lengths. J Physiol 517(Pt 3):831–837

Chapter 8

Pressure Myography

Lars Jørn Jensen

Abstract

Vasomotor function (constriction, dilation) can be assessed ex vivo using the pressure myograph technique, also referred to as perfusion myography in older literature. The technique involves isolating an artery (or any other blood vessel/lymphatic vessel) from an animal research model or from surgery-resected human tissue. The vessel preparation is mounted between two tiny glass pipettes through which a physiological saline solution (usually Krebs') is perfused while superfusing the preparation with the same solution. The inner and outer diameter of the vessel can be measured in real time, giving valuable information about the vessel reactivity in response to various vasoconstrictor or vasodilator stimuli in different research models or treatments. In addition, by measuring the passive (100% relaxed) inner and outer diameters of the vessel, important structural information is obtained, which is used to assess the degree of structural remodeling in a disease model or treatment. This technique is not a high-throughput technique and requires highly dedicated and trained personnel to carry out experiments. The reward, however, is highly physiologically relevant data, which can be used to assess the vascular function/dysfunction in almost any vascularized tissue of any human disease model.

Key words Pressure myograph, Perfusion myograph, Arteriole, Resistance artery, Vascular tone, Myogenic tone, Flow-mediated vasodilation, Vascular structural remodeling, Blood pressure, Blood flow

1 Introduction

The mean arterial blood pressure (MAP) and distribution of blood flow in the body are under strict influence by small arteries and arterioles (henceforth "resistance arteries") that can adapt their diameter to changes in physiological conditions and demands. The so-called basal vascular tone is primarily set by the myogenic reactivity of the resistance arteries. Myogenic tone is constantly modulated by input via endothelial dilators (such as shear stress/NO, PGI_2, H_2O_2, and endothelium-dependent hyperpolarization) and sympathetic nerve activity via the release of noradrenaline (plus ATP and NPY) in varicosities on the surface of the smooth muscle layer in the vascular wall. In the longer term, structural remodeling

Dhananjie N. K. Chandrasekera and Rajesh Katare (eds.), *Cardiomyocytes: Methods and Protocols*, Methods in Molecular Biology, vol. 2894, https://doi.org/10.1007/978-1-0716-4342-6_8,

plays an important role in adapting the vessel structure to physiological changes or disease conditions, such as chronic changes in pressure or flow. These are the classical physiological mechanisms that exist in all resistance arteries; however, a multitude of other mechanisms may contribute to vascular tone regulation in a manner that depends on the vascular bed, species, age, sex, and disease conditions. In order to study myogenic tone, flow- and shear stress-mediated vasodilation, and structural remodeling, it is imperative to use an ex vivo technique in which the vessel lumen is perfused and kept under normal physiological pressure that distends the vessels to attain similar dimensions (i.e., wall stress) as if it was in vivo. Pressure myography is such an ex vivo technique. Alternative methods exist in which resistance arteries are surgically exposed and studied in vivo during anesthesia (so-called intravital microscopy), but with such a technique, the experimenter cannot control the pressure and flow in the lumen of the vessel, nor is there a direct access to the abluminal or luminal side for exposure to agonists and antagonists. Furthermore, as with any in vivo technique, the anesthetic agents may interfere with the vascular reactivity under study. There are recent excellent reviews explaining the theory and importance of the pressure myograph technique [1, 2]. The present paper is a comprehensive description of the experimental setup, preparations, and procedures enabling an investigator to initiate and attain experimental routine using this powerful technique. Thus, the paper contains an outline of (1) the materials and equipment needed, (2) how to set up and prepare a pressure myograph experiment, (3) how to dissect a resistance artery from different organs and species, (4) how to mount the vessels in the pressure myograph, and (5) how to perform the initial experimental procedures in order to confirm vessel viability and reactivity. With no doubt, there will be areas that are not covered, but this chapter should enable researchers from all areas of physiology or medicine to carry out their first pressure myograph experiments, provided they have access to suitable equipment and space.

2 Materials

2.1 Buffers

All physiological buffers must be prepared with ultrapure water (resistivity 18.2 MΩ·cm^2 at 25 °C), and all chemicals, reagents, should be analytical grade (≥95% purity) and if possible cell culture tested.

1. Modified Krebs–Henseleit solution (KHS; *see* **Note 1**), composition: NaCl 118 mmol/L, KCl 4.7 mmol/L, $MgSO_4$ 1.2 mmol/L, $CaCl_2{\cdot}2H_2O$ 2 mmol/L, $NaHCO_3$ 25 mmol/L, KH_2PO_4 1.2 mmol/L, D-(+)-glucose 5 mmol/L. *See* **Note 2**.

2. Ca^{2+}-free modified KHS: same as above but with 2 mmol/L EGTA replacing $CaCl_2 \cdot 2H_2O$. Add glucose and equilibrate with CO_2 as for KHS. *See* **Note 3**.
3. High-KCl modified KHS (K75): NaCl 49, KCl 73.7 mmol/L, $MgSO_4$ 1.2 mmol/L, $CaCl_2 \cdot 2H_2O$ 2 mmol/L, $NaHCO_3$ 25 mmol/L, KH_2PO_4 1.2 mmol/L, D-(+)-glucose 5 mmol/L. Add glucose and equilibrate with CO_2 as for KHS.
4. 11 mM-KCl modified KHS (K11): NaCl 112.9 mmol/L, KCl 9.8 mmol/L, $MgSO_4$ 1.2 mmol/L, $CaCl_2 \cdot 2H_2O$ 2 mmol/L, $NaHCO_3$ 25 mmol/L, KH_2PO_4 1.2 mmol/L, D-(+)-glucose 5 mmol/L. Add glucose and equilibrate with CO_2 as for KHS.
5. Mounting buffer—nominally Ca^{2+}-free HEPES-buffered PSS: NaCl 140 mmol/L, KCl 5 mmol/L, $MgCl_2 \cdot 6H_2O$ 1.2 mmol/L, HEPES 10 mmol/L, Mannitol 6 mmol/L, D-(+)-glucose 5 mmol/L. Adjust pH to 7.4 at RT using concentrated NaOH (1 or 2 mol/L). Add glucose (0.5 mL/100 mL) from a 1 mol/L stock solution immediately before use. Do not equilibrate with CO_2.
6. BSA (low endotoxin, cell culture tested). Stock solutions of vasoactive agonists (hormones/peptides, vasoconstrictors, or vasodilators) and antagonists (small molecules, peptides, or antibodies) (*see* **Note 4**).
7. Pressurized gas cylinders with pressure-reducing valves. Cylinders should contain either O_2/CO_2 mixture (5% CO_2, 95% O_2) or air mixture with CO_2 (5% CO_2, 21% O_2, balance N_2). Connect the pressure reducing valves to a system of tubes for dividing the gas mixtures into at least four to five different glass containers with modified KHS of various compositions. A gas distribution manifold is convenient as it can divide the feeding gas line into several parallel lines and is equipped with a stop cock on each line. At the end of each gas tube, place a small diffuser ("bubble stone"), made of an inert material such as metal or hard plastic that can be autoclaved.

2.2 Equipment

1. Pressure myograph system: pressure myograph (such as DMT models 110P, 111P, 114P, 120CP, and 202CM; Living Systems model CH-1), flowmeter (optional); inverted high-quality light microscope with 5–10× objectives (optionally an inverted epifluorescence microscope, such as Olympus IX 71), in-line solution heater with automatic temperature controller, dual-channel peristaltic pump, pressure- and chemical-resistant pump tubing (such as Cole Parmer C-FLEX® or PHARMED® BPT Tubing), silicone tubing (1 × 3 mm and 1.5 × 3 mm) for pressure myograph and superfusion line.

2. Dissection platform: High-quality stereo microscope with adjustable (zoom) magnification from 7.5–60× (such as Leica M80) with ergonomic binocular or trinocular (camera port; *see* **Note 5**) tube; a heavy-based swing-arm stand or table/wall-mounted swingflex-arm for stereo microscope, cold light source (such as LED) with two-arm combination light guide for reflected light (avoid objective-mounted ring-shaped lamp; *see* **Note 6**).
3. Glass pipette fabrication platform: Pipette puller (such as Sutter P-30, P-97, or P-2000), pipette beveler (such as Sutter BV-10; Narishige EG-45 or EG-402), Microforge (such as Narishige MF-830/MF-2).
4. Accessories: calibration shunt (two 10 cm 1.5 × 3 mm silicone tubes connected via a 2 cm hard PVC tubing with a 150–200 μm bore), borosilicate glass capillaries—standard wall (o.d. 1.2 mm, i.d. 0.69 mm, length 100 mm), diamond glass cutter, stage micrometer, fine grinding stone and oil (to sharpen dissection tools), two pairs (four) fine micro-forceps (such as Dumont #5), spring scissors (curved, 8–10 mm blade length), ophthalmic scissors (straight, 4–5 mm blade length), bone cutter (straight or slightly curved, 8 mm blade), small metal spatula (rounded, flat), sharp scalpel, glass Petri dish with black Sylgard® bottom for general dissections (Ø10 cm, depth 1 cm), small deep glass dish with black Sylgard® bottom for brain dissections (Ø 4–5 cm, depth 2–3 cm), insect pins, wooden 10–15 cm cotton swabs, glass dish (Ø 2.5 cm, depth 0.5 cm) with painted black bottom for vessel trimming, 5 mL Luer-Lock syringe, 33 mm syringe filter (0.2 μm), 40 μm tungsten wire, 11/0 nylon suture.

3 Methods

The following procedures are detailed for use with a pressure myograph (*see* **Note 7**) having pressure transducers installed on either side of the myograph chamber and pipettes (*see* **Note 8**), with the pressure head delivered via a 500 mL bluecap flask connected with a pipette on either side of the myograph chamber (e.g., DMT model 120CP). In this type of myograph, intraluminal flow can be turned off completely, or it can be induced by a pressure difference (ΔP) between the two pipettes. Alternatively, the procedures can be performed using a simpler pressure myograph without pressure transducers, in which the intraluminal pressure is controlled via an electronic pressure regulator ("air pump") via two 25 mL bluecap flask on either side of the myograph bath and pipettes (e.g., DMT model 202CM). In this simpler setup, the intraluminal flow can be adjusted via the height difference (gravitational ΔP) between the two flasks being pressurized by the electronic pressure regulator.

3.1 Preparing the Myograph for an Experiment

1. Start by filling the 500 mL bluecap flask with 250–300 mL of KHS, and insert it in the perfusion line on the incoming pressure side of the myograph (P1, right side). Insert an empty 500 mL bluecap flask in the perfusion line on the outcoming pressure side of the myograph (P2, left side). Check that the glass bottleneck and thread are 100% intact. There must be no cracks felt by the touch of your fingertips. Tighten the bluecap lids with the pressure tubing in place on the incoming and outgoing sides of the myograph.
2. Open the pressure source to establish a feeding pressure of 0.25–0.5 mbar in the back of the pressure regulator with the P1 and P2 flasks.
   (i) Check that the three-way valves on the myograph are positioned so that incoming pressure from P1 goes into the glass pipette (*see* **Note 8**) on the right side and outgoing pressure goes into P2 flask on the left side.
   (ii) To flush the myograph perfusion line with KHS, disconnect the pipettes from the pressure line, and connect the right and left side pressure transducers directly using a short piece of pressure tubing with a "dummy vessel" (calibration shunt) inserted in the middle. This calibration shunt mimics the resistance offered by a small artery.
   (iii) Using the pressure interface or your myograph software, set the P1 pressure to 150 mm Hg and the P2 pressure to 70 mm Hg (remember to enable intraluminal flow in interface or software).
   (iv) Start the pressure controller and observe that KHS is drawn from the P1 flask into the perfusion line filling the calibration shunt and finally dripping into the P2 flask. Make sure that P1 and P2 pressures are stable around 150 and 70 mm Hg, respectively.
   (v) Continue flushing for at least 15 min, and make sure that all air bubbles are flushed out of the perfusion line. The myograph chamber and the perfusion tubing may be gently tapped using your fingers to loosen air bubbles that may be stuck in the tubing.
3. Now lower the set P1 and P2 pressures to 70 mm Hg and observe that P1 and P2 pressures stabilize at the desired values.
   (i) Then lower the P2 pressure to 60 mm Hg, still with flow enabled, and observe that both pressures remain stable in time (P1 = 70 mm Hg; P2 = 60 mm Hg).

(ii) Now, disable intraluminal flow by closing the P2 perfusion line between the myograph and the P2 flask (done in the interface or software), and you should observe that the P2 pressure tracks the pressure in the P1 pressure transducer (P1 = 70 mm Hg; "new" P2 = 70 mm Hg). If not, the pressure calibration is inaccurate and must be repeated until you can perform the above procedure (70/60 mm Hg, no flow) with the correct outcome.

(iii) When done, enable the flow again and slowly flush the myograph for a short while at the 70/60 mm Hg pressure difference. Now it is time to connect the pipettes with the pressure transducers and the perfusion line (see next step).

4. Place the myograph in front of you on a flat surface where you can observe the myograph chamber and pipettes using a stereo microscope (usually your dissection platform). When you move the myograph from the stage of the microscope to the tabletop, please enable the pressure regulator and the intraluminal flow, such that large pressure fluctuations are avoided.

   (i) Set the pressure to a low value of your choice (e.g., 20–40 mm Hg).

   (ii) Now stop the pressure regulator and shut the perfusion lines on either side of the myograph using the three-way valves.

   (iii) The pressure calibration shunt may now be removed without pushing buffer out of the system.

   (iv) Fill the myograph bath with 7–8 mL mounting buffer, thereby submerging both pipette tips in the buffer.

   (v) Use a 5–10 mL syringe with a 16–18 gauge needle (cut the needle halfway to remove the tip) to draw mounting buffer into each pipette with attached silicone tubing using manual suction.

   (vi) Mount the silicone tubing to connect both pipettes to the respective inlets toward the P1 and P2 pressure transducers. Open the three-way valves again and observe that buffer is being pushed from the perfusion line into the pipettes.

5. It is recommended to fill the myograph perfusion line and pipettes with KHS containing 1% BSA to mimic physiological conditions.

   (i) From a volume of KHS equilibrated with a 5% CO_2 gas mixture, pour 20 mL KHS into a glass beaker and drizzle 0.2 g of BSA onto the surface. Cover the beaker with Parafilm® and wait for the BSA to dissolve by itself (do not stir).

(ii) When dissolved, draw 4 mL of the 1% BSA/KHS into a 5 mL syringe, mount a 33 mm sterile filter, and press the buffer out until all air has been removed from the filter.

(iii) Mount a short (5 cm) silicone pressure tube (1 × 3 mm) on the sterile filter using a 16–18 gauge needle with the tip cut away.

(iv) Repeat procedure on a second syringe/sterile filter/ pressure tube.

(v) Withdraw about 1 cm air into the tip of each pressure tube and mount them on the three-way valves on the P1 and P2 side of the myograph bath.

(vi) Open the three-way valves to allow flow from the syringe toward the pressure transducers and pipettes on the P1 and P2 sides.

(vii) Carefully, press the 1% BSA/KHS through the sterile filter into the P1 side through the pressure transducer and the pipette. During this delicate step, take great care that the pressure reading from the P1 pressure transducer under no instance exceeds 200 mm Hg (try to keep it under 150 mm Hg).

(viii) Observe that the 1 cm air bubble is slowly advancing through the perfusion line and eventually through the pipette tip into the bath. This ensures that the pipettes and perfusion line within the myograph are filled with the BSA solution.

(ix) Repeat the previous step on the P2 side to fill this pipette with 1% BSA/KHS.

(x) Keep the three-way valves in that position until you have mounted a blood vessel between the P1 and P2 pipettes in the bath.

3.2 Dissecting and Trimming a Blood Vessel Before Mounting in the Myograph

1. *Rat mesenteric small arteries* (fifth order, ~150 μm relaxed lumen diameter) with myogenic reactivity are straightforward to dissect, prepare, and mount and are therefore recommended for those about to learn this technique. Alternatively, use mouse second–fourth-order mesenteric arteries. *See* **Note 9**.

   (i) In brief: after euthanizing the rat or mouse, the abdominal wall should be cut open across and lengthwise, and the intestines should be removed including the cecum (cut below the stomach and above the rectum).

   (ii) Place the intestines in a beaker of CO_2-equilibrated KHS at room temperature. If you are working fast, no ice cooling will be necessary, and in some experiments, initial cooling will even destroy the physiological responses.

(iii) Fill a Petri dish with Sylgard® bottom halfway up with CO_2-equilibrated KHS and transfer the intestines into it while taking care not to move feces or hair along with it.

(iv) Using cotton swabs, spread out the small intestine with the longest loop upward to the left (9–12 o'clock) and secure it with insect pins making sure that it is stretched out, but not overstretched. In this arrangement, usually the arteries are facing upward, and veins are facing downward in the transparent mesentery.

(v) Using curved spring scissors, remove the fatty cartilage structure covering the entry of the large mesenteric artery (zero and first order) toward the distal vessels.

(vi) Now the artery should be visible as filled with bright red blood (not darkish/bluish color as in the vein). Arteries are furthermore distinguishable from veins by having a white, muscular wall (which is not discernable in veins) and the branching points are Y-shaped, not U-shaped as in veins.

(vii) Using sharpened fine micro-forceps and a pair of fine ophthalmic scissors, grip and lift the fat or connective tissue above an artery while cutting with the scissors in parallel to and as close as possible to the vessel wall. When you release the grip in the tissue, you should see that the vessel wall on the upper side is now free from fat and connective tissue.

(viii) Now grip the fat/connective tissue on the lower side of the same artery and repeat the parallel cut with the scissors. If done correctly, the artery should now be completely free from connective tissue and fat.

(ix) Continue this process along the vessel tree until you have reached the segment of your interest. *See* **Note 10**.

(x) Each branch may be cut away and removed when sufficiently long (0.5–1 cm) for your experiments. *See* **Note 11**.

(xi) The entire procedure is the same for mouse mesenteric arteries, with minor modifications due to size differences.

(xii) Store the excised mesenteric artery segments at room temperature in a small glass dish filled with 1% BSA/KHS for further trimming and until mounting in the myograph. *See* **Note 12**.

(xiii) See examples of pressure myograph-mounted mouse and rat mesenteric arteries in Figs. 1 and 2.

2. *Rat and mouse middle cerebral arteries* (MCA) are often used for pressure myograph experiments and are straightforward to isolate and mount in the pressure myograph because, like

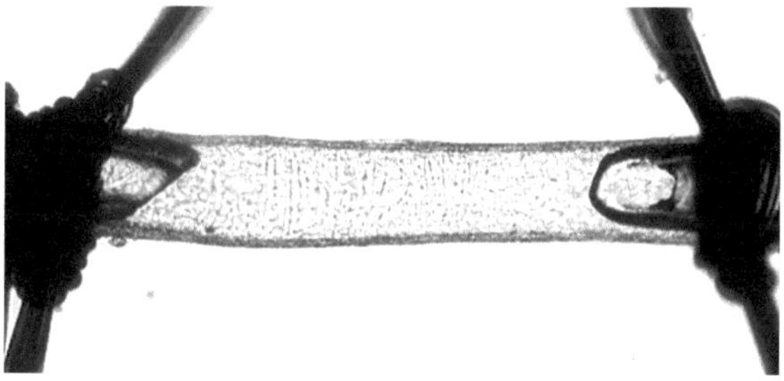

Fig. 1 Mouse mesenteric artery mounted in pressure myograph. Pipette tip outer diameter ~ 80 μm; pressure 40 mm Hg; superfused with Krebs' buffer, 5 mM glucose, 5% CO_2/95% O_2; lumen perfused with Krebs' buffer + 1% BSA. (Data from Björling et al. [3])

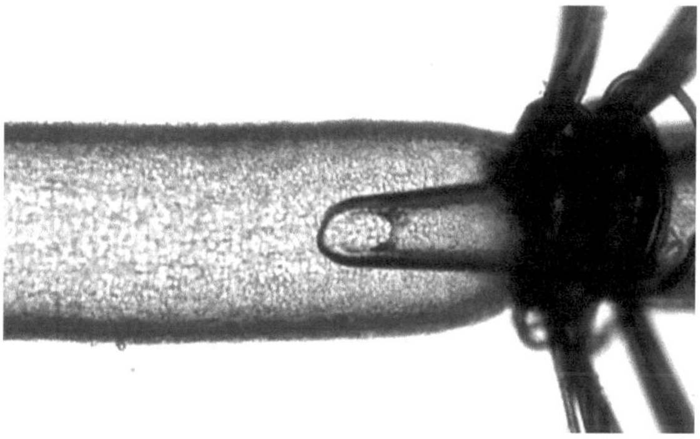

Fig. 2 Rat mesenteric artery mounted in pressure myograph. Pipette tip outer diameter ~ 80 μm; pressure 60 mm Hg; superfused with Krebs' buffer, 5 mM glucose, 5% CO_2/95% O_2; lumen perfused with Krebs' buffer + 1% BSA. (Data from Mikkelsen et al. [4])

mesenteric arteries, they have few side branches. The mouse MCAs are rather small (70–80 μm) and may be difficult to mount between the pipettes for some investigators. The isolation procedures for rat and mouse MCAs are essentially the same.

(i) Start by removing the head from the animal and remove the skin from the head as much as possible.

(ii) While holding the head in one hand, use a small size bone cutter (see Subheading 2.2, **item 4**) to open the upper side of the skull along the midline. Use the tip of the bone cutter to break and remove the skull on either side of the cut.

(iii) Now use a flat, rounded metal object such as a spatula to insert under the brain along the sides of the remaining skull. Gently lift away the brain while making sure to sever the attachments between the brain and the skull underneath in the process. Use only gentle force, as the brain is fragile, especially around the olfactory bulb and the brain stem.

(iv) Transfer the brain to a deep glass Petri dish with Sylgard® bottom and use a sharp scalpel to gently cut the entire brain into a left and a right side.

(v) The two brain halves can now be fixed with the cut side facing downward using small insect needles.

(vi) The middle cerebral artery should be distinguishable at the surface of the brain as a thin vessel with bright red color and a white wall, covered with transparent pial membrane. The brain halves may be tilted to keep the vessel in focus during the isolation procedure.

(vii) Use the sharpened micro-forceps and a pair of ophthalmic scissors to gently excise the MCA without stretching while taking great care to remove as much pial membrane as possible in the process.

(viii) See examples of pressure myograph-mounted rat middle cerebral arteries in Fig. 3a, b.

3. *Porcine intramural left coronary small arteries* (second–third-generation branches from LCA) are suited for pressure myography as they are ~200–400 μm in diameter and have less dense branching than the deeper, smaller intramural coronary arteries.

A B

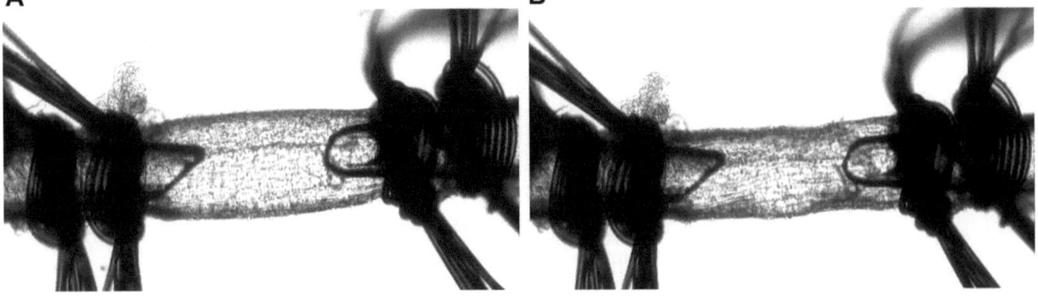

Fig. 3 (**a**, **b**) Rat middle cerebral artery mounted in pressure myograph. Pipette tip outer diameter ~ 80 μm; pressure 40 mm Hg (**a**, without tone); pressure 100 mm Hg (**b**, with myogenic tone); superfused with Krebs' buffer, 5 mM glucose, 5% CO_2/95% O_2; lumen perfused with Krebs' buffer + 1% BSA. (Unpublished)

(i) Start by excising the heart from the euthanized pig and transfer it on ice to the laboratory.

(ii) The dissection is carried out under the stereo microscope in a Petri dish placed on ice in a flat tray. *See* **Note 13**.

(iii) Using the sharpened micro-forceps and a pair of curved spring scissors, cut the heart muscle away along the descending LAD and follow its diagonal branches as far as possible as they run into the left myocardium and dive deeper into the tissue and become intramuscular small arteries.

(iv) From this point, use only the micro-forceps and a pair of small ophthalmic scissors. Gently cut away as much heart muscle as possible from the small arteries diving deep into the ventricular tissue, taking care not to stretch or poke the vessels.

(v) Once a segment of 0.5 cm length is cleaned, cut away and place it in a small glass dish filled with ice-cold 1% BSA/KHS.

(vi) If necessary before mounting in the pressure myograph, the vessels may be trimmed by removing excess fat, muscle, and connective tissue. *See* **Note 14**.

(vii) See example of pressure myograph-mounted porcine coronary artery branch in Fig. 4.

4. *Porcine small pial arteries* (100–200 μm) are well suited for pressure myograph studies being sufficiently long without branching and small enough to possess strong myogenic reactivity.

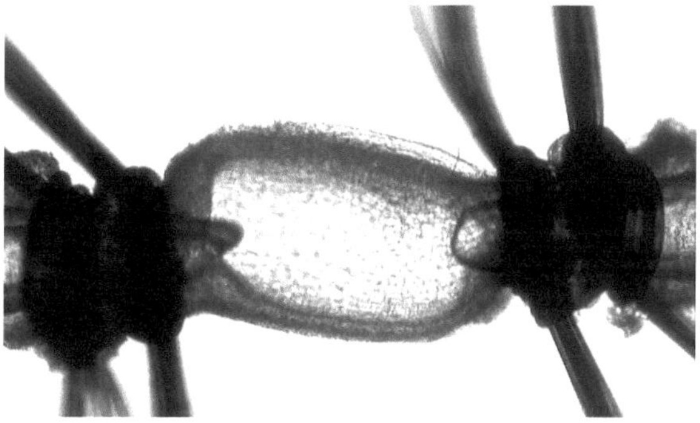

Fig. 4 Göttingen minipig left coronary artery intramural branch (second or third order), mounted in pressure myograph. Pipette tip outer diameter ~ 100 μm; pressure 100 mm Hg; superfused with Ca^{2+}-free Krebs' buffer (i.e. passive), 5 mM glucose, 5% CO_2/95% O_2; lumen perfused with Krebs' buffer + 1% BSA. (Data from Boonen et al. [5])

- (i) Start by cutting the head away from the euthanized minipig or young landrace (farm) pig weighing no more than 80–100 kg.
- (ii) The head should be immediately halved using a bandsaw or transported quickly on ice to a place where this can be done.
- (iii) The half head is placed with the brain facing upward, and using two flat, rounded metal spoons or spatulas, the brain may be gently removed from inside its cavity.
- (iv) Each brain half should be quickly transferred to a beaker with ice-cold CO_2-equilibrated KHS and immediately transported to the Lab. *See* **Note 1**.
- (v) The following isolation procedures may take time, so keep the beakers with the brain halves on ice.
- (vi) Place one brain half in a large glass dish and cut away areas of interest for further dissections using a sharp scalpel.
- (vii) Place a piece of brain tissue containing several pial arteries on the surface under the stereo microscope. The pial arteries are distinguished from the veins due to their bright red color and white walls.
- (viii) Using the sharpened micro-forceps and ophthalmic scissors, peel away pial membrane around a small artery diving into the fissures in the cortex of the brain.
- (ix) While holding the proximal end of the small artery with the forceps, gently cut away pial membrane around the more distal branches of the pial arterial tree.
- (x) At this anatomical position, the brain tissue is quite soft, and in our experience, gently teasing the distal branches of the arteries away from the brain tissue does not damage their structure or function.
- (xi) Once a sufficiently long (0.5–2 cm) arterial tree with pial branches is free from brain tissue, cut the distal end and transfer the vessels to a small glass dish for trimming.
- (xii) Select a suitable small pial artery branch for pressure myography and remove any brain tissue (*see* **Note 15**) and as much pial membrane as possible.
- (xiii) See example of pressure myograph-mounted porcine small pial artery branch in Fig. 5.

5. *Porcine terminal mesenteric arteries* (200–500 μm).
   - (i) From the omental circulation (mesentery) along the small intestine, excise a segment of approx. 10–15 cm in length at a pre-defined location (e.g., 40–50 cm proximally/orally to the cecum).

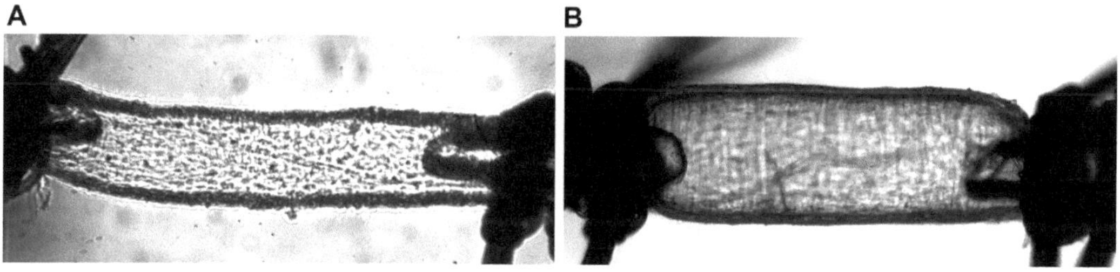

Fig. 5 (**a**, **b**) Göttingen minipig pial (cerebral) arteries mounted in pressure myograph. Pipette tip outer diameter ~ 80 μm and pressure 60 mm Hg in both arteries. Small pial branch with myogenic tone (**a**) and another larger passive/relaxed branch (**b**). Superfused with Krebs' buffer (**a**) or Ca^{2+}-free Krebs' buffer (**b**), 5 mM glucose, 5% CO_2/95% O_2; lumen perfused with Krebs' buffer + 1% BSA. (Data from Björling et al. [3] (**a**) and Ludvigsen et al. [6] (**b**))

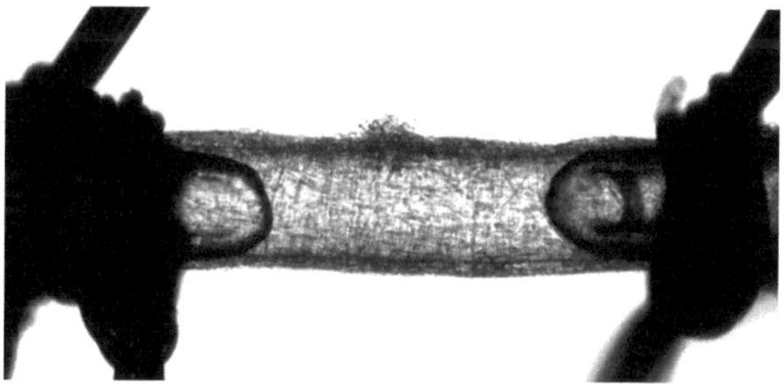

Fig. 6 Newborn piglet terminal mesenteric artery mounted in pressure myograph. Pipette tip outer diameter ~ 80 μm; pressure 40 mm Hg; superfused with Krebs' buffer, 5 mM glucose, 5% CO_2/95% O_2; lumen perfused with Krebs' buffer + 1% BSA. (Unpublished)

(ii) Locate the terminal branches of the mesenteric arteries (TMA) arranged perpendicularly to the axis of the small intestine and cut away a small piece of tissue with 2–3 TMAs.

(iii) The TMAs run adjacent to the veins emerging from the intestinal wall, and it is necessary to carefully remove or cut open the connective tissue that wraps around both vessels.

(iv) Once this task is accomplished, isolation of a 0.5–2 cm long segment of TMA is straightforward.

(v) See example of pressure myograph-mounted porcine terminal mesenteric arteries in Figs. 6 and 7.

6. Keep the dissected vessels in a glass dish (Ø 2.5 cm, black bottom) filled with freshly O_2/CO_2 equilibrated KHS, glucose, and 1% BSA until use in the pressure myograph. *See* **Note 12**.

Fig. 7 Göttingen minipig terminal mesenteric artery mounted in pressure myograph. Pipette tip outer diameter ~ 80 μm; pressure 60 mm Hg; superfused with Ca^{2+}-free Krebs' buffer (i.e., passive), 5 mM glucose, 5% CO_2/95% O_2; lumen perfused with Krebs' buffer + 1% BSA. (Data from Ludvigsen et al. [6])

3.3 Mounting Small Arteries on Pipettes in the Pressure Myograph

1. Start by placing the glass dish with the dissected vessels under a high-quality stereo microscope.
   (i) Using the tips of your sharpened forceps, turn over each vessel segment gently by pushing or holding onto a piece of connective tissue or adipose tissue near the end of the segments. Take a note of the proximal versus distal ends of each segment. *See* **Note 16**.
   (ii) Select an undamaged segment without any side branches and as clean as possible in the middle of the segment (*see* **Note 17**). In general, only the middle half or one-third of the vessel is being pressurized in the experiment. The rest is being pulled over the pipette tips and secured with suture knots.
   (iii) Transfer the selected vessel segment to another glass dish filled with "mounting buffer" for gentle relaxation of the vessel while handling it. Hold onto some connective tissue at the end of the vessel during transfer (the vessel is not damaged by this short exposure to air). Alternatively, use a glass Pasteur pipette to transfer the segment in a small volume of buffer.
   (iv) Cut a short piece of 40 μm tungsten wire about twice the length of the vessel segment and place it next to the segment in the glass dish.
   (v) The segments are often closed at both ends due to the cut by the ophthalmic scissor. Under the stereo microscope, gently push or pull the vessel ends so that they open. This needs to be done very gently and only by touching the vessel segment at the very ends. Avoid stretching or poking at the vessels at any time, except at the very ends of the segments.

(vi) Next, grab the tungsten wire with a micro-forceps in one hand, and push it into the most proximal part of the vessel while securing the vessel with a micro-forceps in your other hand. This also needs to be done very gently to avoid damaging the endothelium, but in the authors' experience, endothelial damage during this step rarely happens if ever.

(vii) Advance the wire so that the vessel covers the center of the wire, leaving some wire outside the proximal end of the vessel. The segment is now ready for transfer to the pressure myograph chamber.

2. Suture knots are prepared under the stereo microscope as double loops of the ophthalmic 11–0 suture in advance or just before your experiment. Place the pressure myograph bath in front of you under the stereo microscope and push two open suture knots onto the shaft of each pipette. Later, when the double loops are tightened around the vessel, they will lock it in place onto the pipette.

3. Hold onto the exposed tungsten wire at the proximal end of the vessel segment using a micro-forceps, and transfer the vessel from the glass dish into the myograph chamber filled with mounting buffer.

   (i) The proximal vessel end should be mounted onto the P1 pipette tip to ensure the physiological flow direction from the proximal (P1, right) to distal (P2, left) side of the preparation.

   (ii) Under high magnification (~30–50×) in the stereo microscope, adjust focus on the pipette tip so that the opening of the beveled pipette tip is clearly seen. *See* **Note 1**.

   (iii) Have two micro-forceps ready for tightening the suture knots.

   (iv) Zoom out with your left hand on the microscope while grabbing the free end of the wire with the right hand using the micro-forceps. Lift the wire and vessel to a position in front of the P1 pipette tip. With the left hand, zoom in again on the pipette tip as before.

   (v) Now, grab the second micro-forceps with your left hand. Using your left hand, support the right-hand forceps holding the vessel and wire, to minimize any shaking or movements of the wire. Now, slowly advance the end of the wire into the open pipette tip and let go of the wire while making sure it will stay inside the tip.

   (vi) With the right-hand forceps supported by the left-hand forceps to reduce shaking, grab a little connective tissue at the proximal end of the vessel and slowly move it closer to the pipette tip along the wire, and finally let the vessel opening slide over the beveled tip. This must be done in a slow, nonstop, careful movement.

(vii) Put the left forceps down and support your right-hand forceps using the left-hand fingers. Slowly push the proximal end of the vessel further onto the pipette, until about one-third of the isolated segment is on the pipette.

(viii) Under a lower magnification (~20–30×), move one suture knot near the pipette tip and tighten it slightly until only a small loop is left.

(ix) Grab each end of the suture near the double loop and slowly advance the still open loop over the vessel segment covering the pipette tip, as far toward the tip end as possible. Now, in one careful movement, tighten the knot using exactly equal pull force on each side of the loop. Once you feel the knot is tightened, carefully pull a little more using small equally forced movements, to secure the knot.

4. Open the three-way valve to the P1 (right side) pipette to let a passive pressure head push the vessel open and flush any blood out of the vessel.

(i) Using the right-hand forceps, remove the wire carefully not to damage the endothelium. Now close the P1 valve again to stop flushing the vessel.

(ii) Advance the P1 pipette and vessel segment horizontally toward the P2 pipette tip using the millimeter dial on the right side. Make sure that the vessel overlaps a little with the P2 pipette tip.

(iii) Adjust the zoom to high magnification and adjust focus to get a clear view of the P2 pipette tip. The open end of the vessel segment might now be slightly off focus, which can be a challenge.

(iv) Very carefully, using the right hand micro-forceps, with the support of your left hand, grab a snip of loose connective tissue at the end of the vessel segment and move it in front of the P2 pipette tip to be in focus. Using tiny controlled movement, slide the open vessel end onto the pipette tip taking care not to touch the tip or to stretch/pinch the artery. This might take some practice to learn. Once the vessel is on the tip, let go of the vessel with the forceps.

(v) Adjust focus and move the P1 pipette a little closer to the P2 pipette tip, if necessary. With very controlled movement, push the end of the vessel segment further up onto the pipette until about one-third of the segment is on the pipette. Make sure that any remaining adipose tissue or potential leaks/side branches are on the pipette tip.

(vi) At this point, you can open the three-way valve on the right side shortly to fill the vessel to make sure that it is straight. If twisted, rotate the vessel segment in place by careful adjustment using the tip of your micro-forceps.

(vii) Repeat the tightening of the two suture knots as for the P1 pipette.

5. Any blood stemming from the vessel segment must be dispersed from the bottom of the chamber and removed before starting an experiment (flush using a 1 mL pipette).

(i) With the suture knots in place on P1 and P2 pipettes, open the three-way valves on both sides to allow flow into the vessel.

(ii) Now, activate the myograph pressure controller to set a pressure of 40 mm Hg in both pipettes, and start the heating of the myograph chamber (typically to 37 °C).

(iii) You should see the vessel being pressurized with full visibility of the lumen and the vessel wall along the entire segment.

(iv) If necessary, stretch the vessel segment by retracting the P1 pipette horizontally to the right, to avoid bending of the segment.

(v) Check that there are no leaks, which would be visible as buffer with BSA being pushed out of the vessel (looks like cloudy or hazy fluid near the vessel). If you have a big leak or side branch, a new vessel segment must be mounted as otherwise the pressure drop will be too high during an experiment.

3.4 Starting a Pressure Myograph Experiment

1. With the pressure controller activated at a pressure of 40 mm Hg (to prevent excessive pressure fluctuations), lift the myograph chamber and slowly transfer it to the stage of your microscope.

(i) In the software, activate the camera view and adjust the microscope focus and light until the vessel lumen and walls become clearly visible. The background should be nearly white (brightly lit) and the vessel walls should appear as dark as possible. The lumen should be brighter than the vessel walls and clearly distinguishable.

(ii) Now make a rectangle (ROI) in the software covering the middle part of the pressurized vessel segment. The software's diameter measurements should be clearly tracking the inner and outer boundaries of the vessel segment, respectively. The larger the ROIs are, the more stable the diameter measurements are.

(iii) In pressure steps of 20 mm Hg, slowly increase the pressure in both pipettes until the highest pressure to be used in your experiment (e.g., 120 mm Hg). During this procedure, stretch the vessel segment using the P1 pipette millimeter dial until the vessel is not bending and is slightly stretched out. Stretch only until the point where the vessel segment begins to change its shape around the ends.

(iv) At the highest pressure, disable the flow in the P2 pipette (as in a blind sac experiment) and observe the pressure reading in both pipettes. If no leak, the pressures should be similar.

(v) If a small leak is present, the pressure on the P2 side might drop 2–3 mm Hg. This is not a problem if you run your experiment with flow enabled in the P2 pipette, so that pressure inside the vessel lumen is maintained constant.

(vi) If the leak is larger and the P2 pressure drops 5 mm Hg or more, it might be a problem to keep the vessel pressurized and responsive for an entire experiment.

(vii) Assuming that there are no major leaks, lower the pressure to your desired value (e.g., 60 mm Hg) and remember to start recording of your data.

(viii) Finally, start gas bubbling (O_2/CO_2) of the chamber via a steel pipe in the myograph lid.

2. At this point, the author prefers to use a standard protocol in all pressure myograph experiments to check the vitality of the smooth muscle and endothelial functions. After that, your desired protocol for the particular experiment can be performed. A standard protocol might be as follows:

   (i) Superfuse with high-KCl KHS (e.g., 75 mM KCl) to monitor depolarization-induced constriction. The constriction should come fast (not just transiently), be powerful (closing or almost closing the vessel lumen), and be uniform along the entire length of the vessel segment. Wash out with normal KHS after 4–5 min, and allow the vessel to come back to the baseline diameter.

   (ii) Wait at least 5 min before superfusing with a submaximal concentration of noradrenaline (1 μM) in KHS. The constriction might be slower, but at steady-state, the constriction should be at least 20% and uniform along the entire vessel segment.

   (iii) Now, stop the superfusion flow and add a maximal dilating concentration of acetylcholine (10 μM) directly into the bath. The vessel should dilate at least 30%, rapidly and uniformly along the entire vessel segment.

(iv) Wash out noradrenaline and acetylcholine with fresh KHS and wait for baseline diameter to be achieved. Increase pressure in both pipettes by 40 mm Hg (e.g., from 60 to 100 mm Hg) and let the vessel precondition to the higher pressure for 25–30 min. In this time interval, you should see some myogenic tone develop after an initial passive dilation caused by the pressure increase.

3. Now your vessel is ready for your own protocol to start, as you have confirmed the presence of smooth muscle contraction, endothelium-dependent dilation, and myogenic tone.

4 Notes

1. Artificial cerebrospinal fluid (ACSF) may be used during isolation of and experiments with small brain (penetrating or parenchymal) arterioles.
2. Dissolve all salts except $CaCl_2$ in nearly final volume, and then add $CaCl_2$ (2 mL/L) from a 1 mol/L stock solution and top up to final volume. Just before use, add glucose (0.5 mL/100 mL) from a 1 mol/L stock solution. Allow solution to equilibrate with a gas mixture containing 5% CO_2 at least 20 min before use in experiments, and if possible check that pH is 7.4 under your experimental conditions (i.e., in pressure myograph chamber). The KHS without glucose can be stored up to 1 month at 4 °C, but after adding glucose, use it within a day.
3. For large, thick-walled vessels, such as coronary, skeletal muscle, or large cerebral arteries, add L-type channel blocker nifedipine (5 μmol/L) to the Ca^{2+}-free KHS, to completely relax the arteries.
4. In general, these can be dissolved in ultrapure H_2O, PBS, or DMSO at the highest concentration feasible. Make sure that the solvent concentration does not exceed 0.1% in the final solution after adding a substance. Small molecules and some peptides may be stored for several months up to 1 year at −20 ° C. However, the storage property must be experimentally verified for each individual substance tested. The author's Lab has good experience with keeping the most common vasoactive agonists (noradrenaline, acetylcholine, bradykinin, endothelin-1, thromboxane A_2 mimetic U46619, ATP, UTP) for up to 1 year at −20 °C. As a precaution, however, store any substance with unknown storage properties in stock solution for less than 2 months at −20 °C or − 80 °C.

5. A camera port and video monitor may be convenient for demonstrating to students and technical staff how the microdissections should be practically carried out.
6. The latter type of objective-mounted lamp, in the author's experience, causes a halo of light reflections from the surface of the buffer and preparation and is therefore unpractical for microdissections.
7. The pressure myograph should be correctly set up and pressure-calibrated before use (see the myograph user manual). The layout of the myograph, microscope, glass containers for physiological saline solutions, and gas equilibration tubes/diffusers should be conveniently arranged to facilitate a smooth operation. The microscope for dissection and mounting vessels in the myograph should be next to the microscope stage (within 1–2 m). In this way, the myograph chamber does not need to be disconnected from the pressure tubing while mounting the vessels. This greatly reduces problems with air bubbles in the perfusion line.
8. Pull P1 and P2 pipettes using the pipette puller (see Subheading 2.2, **item 3**) and select a program for making a patch-clamp pipette. Make sure that the shank of the pipette is sufficiently long and straight for securing the suture knots. However, the shank should not be too long and thin as this increases the pipette resistance and the risk of clogging the tips. Mount a pipette in the Microforge and manually break down the tip to 20–50 μm in diameter. Now mount the pipette in the beveler, and carefully grind the tip at an angle of approx. 45° until the diameter is suited for the type of vessel you will use. Finally, heat-polish the beveled tips using the Microforge. In general, tip outer diameters from 80 to 120 μm work well with the vessels suggested in the "Methods" section. Make sure that the tip diameters (i.e., resistances) are matched on either side of the vessels in your experiment, to avoid an uneven pressure drop across the pipette tips.
9. Larger branches of rat mesenteric arteries may be used for agonist-induced responses and pharmacology, but do not expect them to develop any myogenic tone. Mouse mesenteric arteries are shorter and smaller than their rat counterparts are, but second- to fourth-order mouse arteries (220–100 μm) are suited for pressure myography, as they do possess myogenic reactivity.
10. You may also start the dissection further down the mesenteric arterial tree to focus on the more distal branches of your interest.

11. In this way, you will get smaller and larger mesenteric artery branches, and the ones that are not used for pressure myograph experiments may be preserved for other experiments.
12. The vessels may also be transferred to the refrigerator if placed in the 1% BSA/KHS with glucose (O_2/CO_2 equilibrated) inside a small glass cylinder with airtight lid. Here they will stay fresh and responsive to physiological stimuli for many hours.
13. Ice is recommended as the heart muscle has a high metabolism, which may affect the coronary arteries if the surrounding muscle becomes anoxic.
14. It is sufficient if the lumen of the vessel is visible in the middle portion of the coronary vessel; however, large tissue chunks may not be present toward the ends, as it prevents tightening the sutures on the glass pipettes during the mounting procedure.
15. It is mandatory to remove all brain tissue around the vessels because it may interfere with your experiments.
16. Note the proximal and distal ends of the isolated vessels by leaving a little extra connective or adipose tissue at the proximal vessel end during dissections.
17. The ends of the segment may have a little connective tissue attached, but do not leave perivascular adipose tissue (PVAT) attached, due to the anti-contractile effects of PVAT.

References

1. Wenceslau CF, McCarthy CG, Earley S, England SK, Filosa JA, Goulopoulou S, Gutterman DD, Isakson BE, Kanagy NL, Martinez-Lemus LA, Sonkusare SK, Thakore P, Trask AJ, Watts SW, Webb RC (2021) Guidelines for the measurement of vascular function and structure in isolated arteries and veins. Am J Physiol Heart Circ Physiol 321(1):H77–H111. https://doi.org/10.1152/ajpheart.01021.2020
2. Schubert R, Gaynullina D, Shvetsova A, Tarasova OS (2023) Myography of isolated blood vessels: considerations for experimental design and combination with supplementary techniques. Front Physiol 24(14):1176748. https://doi.org/10.3389/fphys.2023.1176748
3. Björling K, Joseph PD, Egebjerg K, Salomonsson M, Hansen JL, Ludvigsen TP, Jensen LJ (2018) Role of age, Rho-kinase 2 expression, and G protein-mediated signaling in the myogenic response in mouse small mesenteric arteries. Physiol Rep 6(17):e13863. https://doi.org/10.14814/phy2.13863
4. Mikkelsen MF, Björling K, Jensen LJ (2016) Age-dependent impact of $Ca_V3.2$ T-type calcium channel deletion on myogenic tone and flow-mediated vasodilatation in small arteries. J Physiol 594(20):5881–5898. https://doi.org/10.1113/JP271470
5. Boonen HC, Moesgaard SG, Birck MM, Christoffersen BO, Cirera S, Heegaard PM, Højbøge TR, Jensen LJ, Mortensen A, Olsen LH, Sheykhzade M, Tang J, Lykkesfeldt J (2014) Functional network analysis of obese and lean Göttingen minipigs elucidates changes in oxidative and inflammatory networks in obese pigs. Pflugers Arch 466(12):2167–2176. https://doi.org/10.1007/s00424-014-1486-2
6. Ludvigsen TP, Olsen LH, Pedersen HD, Christoffersen BØ, Jensen LJ (2019) Hyperglycemia-induced transcriptional regulation of ROCK1 and TGM2 expression is involved in small artery remodeling in obese diabetic Göttingen Minipigs. Clin Sci (Lond) 133(24):2499–2516. https://doi.org/10.1042/CS20191066

Chapter 9

Langendorff Isolated Heart Perfusion Model for Functional Studies in Mice

Esther U. Asamudo, Yann Huey Ng, and Donald M. Bers

Abstract

The ex vivo isolated heart perfusion model by Oskar Langendorff to resuscitate and maintain the automacity of a heart excised from a mammal was introduced in the late nineteenth century. It has remained an essential technique used for functional studies in cardiovascular research even after over a hundred years. This model provides information on contractility, cardiac rhythm, metabolism, and overall cardiac function. It allows the study of the heart in isolation without the influences of other organs or hormones. It enables the investigation of physiological mechanisms underlying heart function under different conditions with more experimental control than the heart in vivo. This chapter provides an overview of the protocol for the isolated heart perfusion model.

Key words Isolated heart, Langendorff, Perfusion, Buffer, Cardiac function

1 Introduction

The isolated heart perfusion technique has remained at the forefront of cardiovascular research to study heart physiology under controlled conditions. The isolated heart perfusion system enables the study of heart function in isolation of other organ systems and exocrine control [1–4]. This technique involves the isolation of the heart and retrograde perfusion of the excised heart through the aorta to the coronary circulation with buffer solution that mimics the blood plasma content, allowing the heart to contract similarly to the in vivo situation [5]. This retrograde aortic perfusion is opposite to the normal physiologic flow; however, it ensures that the heart receives adequate oxygenation and nutrients and thereby maintains the heart's function ex vivo. The model also offers the opportunity to investigate the effects of drugs on heart function in a controlled environment, making it a valuable tool for drug discovery and development [1, 6, 7]. In the isolated heart experiment, it is possible to control different physiological variables such as

Dhananjie N. K. Chandrasekera and Rajesh Katare (eds.), *Cardiomyocytes: Methods and Protocols*, Methods in Molecular Biology, vol. 2894, https://doi.org/10.1007/978-1-0716-4342-6_9,

oxygenation, temperature, coronary flow, and perfusion pressure. Depending on the type of scientific investigation required, this perfusion system can be operated at constant pressure or constant flow. Constant pressure mode is ideal for experiments where the change in flow is autoregulated by the heart, such as during ischemia and reperfusion (I-R), where the flow is variable depending on the phase of I-R; whereas constant flow mode is used for studying the coronary vascular tone, for instance, during the administration of a drug that regulates vascular tone, at a constant flow rate. With a pump controller, it is possible to switch between constant flow and constant pressure perfusion.

The process of a Langendorff isolated heart preparation involves excision of the heart from the donor animal, cannulation of the heart, and reperfusion with perfusion fluid. The next step depends on the type of experiment, the parameters to be measured, and data to be obtained. In most studies, contractile function is measured and the preferred method is the use of a compliant ventricular balloon inserted into the left ventricle (LV) [8]. The balloons can be commercially purchased (not generally recommended) or custom made from polyethylene food wrap or latex [6]. The properties of the LV balloon should include (a) appropriate size to match the heart size, (b) must be highly flexible to fit the contours of the LV wall, (c) high compliance and nonelastic, and (d) durability [6, 9]. Latex material could be from a condom tip or liquid latex [10]. The method of using liquid latex to make balloon is somewhat more complicated compared to using food wrap. However, latex has better compliance and durability.

The important parameters to be controlled in a Langendorff isolated heart setup include temperature, type of perfusate, coronary flow, end-diastolic pressure, and perfusion temperature, which will affect cardiac function and stability. As an ex vivo preparation, it is pertinent to note that the contractile function of the isolated heart will gradually deteriorate, typically at a rate of 5–10% per hour [2]. This depends on several factors including the species and age of the animal, the skill of the researcher, the content of the perfusion fluid, the type of pharmacological intervention, and the workload of the heart [2]. To correct for baseline cardiac deterioration, time-matched controls are critical for inclusion in the study design. Before commencing a study using isolated heart perfusion, pre-defined exclusion criteria under baseline conditions must be established (*see* Table 1).

Functional studies using isolated heart perfusion has several advantages. It can provide detailed information on cardiac contractility, heart rate, metabolism, and electrophysiology under controlled experimental conditions. Isolated heart preparation allows researchers to investigate the effect of drugs on cardiac function as well as their safety and efficacy prior to use for in vivo experiments. It also allows for reproducibility and several interventions. For

Table 1
Exclusion criteria for Langendorff isolated mouse hearts [1, 11, 12]

Parameter	
Time (excision to perfusion, min)	>3
Coronary flow (mL/min)	<1 or > 5
Arrhythmic events (min)	>3
Heart rate (beats per min)	<300 or > 620
Left ventricular developed pressure (mm Hg)	<60 or > 140

example, the direct endogenous effects of cardiac autonomic response can be investigated by stimulating the isolated heart with sympathomimetic or parasympathomimetic agents in the perfusate. Isolated intact hearts with higher levels of structural and functional integration are also of more physiological relevance when compared to organizational structures such as tissues and cellular fragments. Although the isolated heart perfusion model has several advantages, it presents some challenges. The model requires trained personnel with surgical skills and a highly controlled environment, which must be maintained (i.e., temperature). Isolated hearts are also vulnerable to ambient immune stimuli due to the absence of blood-derived antioxidants and glucocorticosteroids [5]. Additionally, ethical issues must be considered, as with all animal experimentation. Taking all these into consideration, isolated heart perfusion remains a reasonably physiological preparation and a robust tool for cardiovascular research. Here we describe a protocol for the Langendorff isolated heart experiment using small mammalian hearts perfused with modified Krebs–Henseleit buffer.

2 Materials

2.1 Buffers and Preparation

1. Modified Krebs–Henseleit buffer (KHB): 118.5 mM NaCl, 4.7 mM KCl, 1.2 mM $MgSO_4 \cdot 7H_2O$, 1.2 mM $KH_2PO_4 \cdot H_2O$, 25 mM $NaHCO_3$, 11 mM Glucose, 1.5 mM $CaCl_2$ (*see* **Note 1**).
   (a) To prepare 1 L of modified Krebs–Henseleit buffer, in a beaker, add 6.925 g of NaCl, 0.35 g of KCl, 0.296 g of $MgSO_4\,7H_2O$, 0.163 g of $KH_2PO_4 \cdot H_2O$, 2.1 g of $NaHCO_3$, and 1.981 g of glucose. Allow this to mix in a beaker at room temperature. When all the salts have dissolved, slowly add 1.5 mL of 1 M $CaCl_2$ solution and bring to volume (*see* **Note 2**). Adjust the pH of the solution to 7.4. Filter the solution using polyethersulfone membrane, 0.22 μM filter. Bubble this solution with

carbogen gas (95% O_2, 5% CO_2) for at least 15–20 min prior to the beginning of an experiment.

2. Cardioplegic solution: 118.5 mM NaCl, 18.8 mM KCl, 1.2 mM $MgSO_4 \cdot 7H_2O$, 1.2 mM $KH_2PO_4 \cdot H_2O$, 25 mM $NaHCO_3$, 11 mM glucose, 0.5 mM $CaCl_2$.
   (a) To prepare 500 mL of fresh cardioplegic solution, in a beaker, add 3.463 g of NaCl, 0.701 g of KCl, 0.148 g of $MgSO_4 \cdot 7H_2O$, 0.081 g of $KH_2PO_4 \cdot H_2O$, 1.05 g of $NaHCO_3$., 0.991 g of glucose, and 250 μL of $CaCl_2$ 1 M solution. Allow this to mix in a beaker at room temperature. When all the salts have dissolved, adjust pH to 7.4. Bring to volume and filter the solution using polyethersulfone membrane, 0.22 μM filter. Store this solution at 4 °C or on ice until ready to use (*see* **Note 3**).
3. 1 M $CaCl_2$ solution.

2.2 Drugs

1. Heparin.
2. Isoflurane.
3. Oxygen.
4. Saline solution.

2.3 Equipment

1. Spring scissors: length, 12 cm; cutting edge, 14 mm; tip diameter, 0.275 mm, sharp, straight.
2. Fine scissors: length, 10 cm; cutting edge, 14 mm; tip, blunt–blunt, straight.
3. Dumont forceps: length, 11 cm; tip, 0.1 × 0.06 mm, angled 45°, standard.
4. Extra fine Graefe forceps: length, 10 cm; tip width, 0.5 mm; tip dimensions, 0.5 × 0.5 mm, curved.
5. Surgical suture: nonabsorbable braided silk, 4–0.
6. Disposable syringes.
7. Disposable injection needles (20 gauge).
8. Table top vaporizer for isoflurane.
9. Tubing: PE-100.
10. Food wrap.
11. Liquid latex: 33% (w/w).
12. Sewing pin with ball head (3 mm).
13. Polyethersulfone membrane.

2.4 Langendorff System

The Langendorff isolated heart rig setup (*see* Fig. 1):

1. A thermostatically controlled water bath and water circulator.
2. Peristaltic pump.

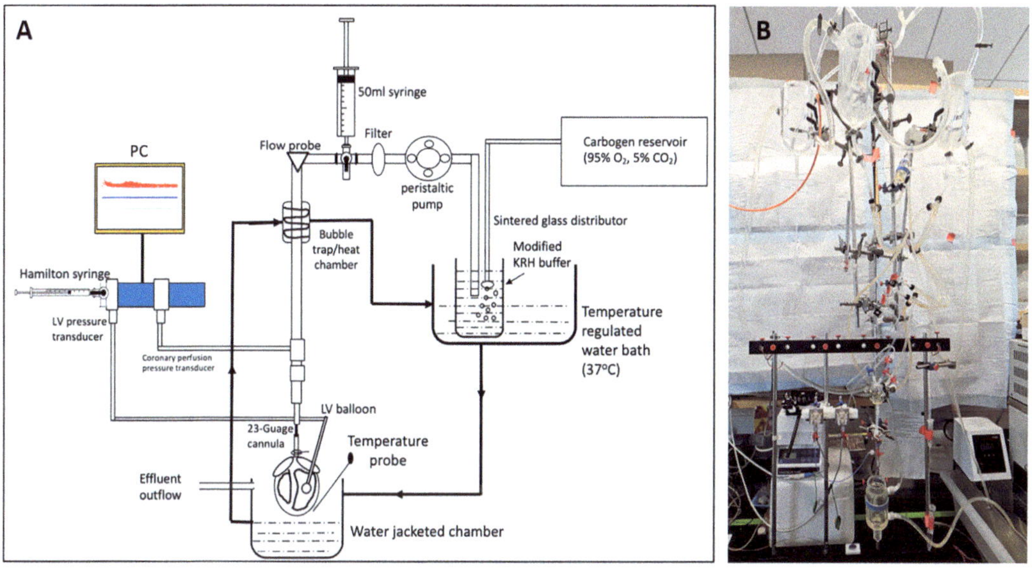

Fig. 1 Langendorff isolated heart setup. (**a**) A mouse heart is cannulated and immersed in an organ bath with a temperature probe to ensure that the temperature is maintained at 37 °C. The flow of the gassed KHB through the system is regulated by a peristaltic pump. The KHB passes through the filter, compliance chamber, the in-line flow probe, the bubble trap/heat chamber, and then into the isolated heart. The pressure transducers are connected to a powerlab equipment which generates signals that are recorded using LabChart software to determine coronary perfusion pressure and LV pressure (connected to the balloon in the left ventricle of the heart). (**b**) Langendorff perfusion setup in the laboratory

3. Pump tubing (3.18 mm, PVC).
4. Flowmeter or in-line flow probe.
5. Pressure pump controller.
6. Pressure transducers (2×) for LV and coronary perfusion pressure.
7. Snap Holder and Bracket for pressure transducers.
8. PowerLab 8/35.
9. Bridge amplifiers (2×).
10. Electrocardiogram (ECG) electrodes.
11. Bubble trap/heat chamber.
12. Compliance chamber.
13. Thermometer or temperature probe.
14. Syringe filter: pore size, 0.45 μm, cellulose acetate membrane; diameter, 33 mm, sterile, FLL/MLL end fitting.
15. Tygon tubing.
16. Double-jacketed heart chamber.
17. Zoom microscope on boom stand: zoom range 0.8–4 × .
18. Carbogen (95% O_2, 5% CO_2).

19. Oxygenators for carbogen.
20. Data acquisition system and analysis software (LabChart or polygraph).

3 Methods

3.1 Perfusion Setup

1. Equilibrate the thermostat water bath temperature to 37 °C (*see* **Note 4**).
2. Place the filtered perfusion solution in the heated water-jacketed reservoir.
3. Place the gas dispersion bubbler into the reservoir containing the perfusion buffer.
4. Turn on the carbogen gas (95% O_2 and 5% CO_2) and continuously oxygenate the perfusion buffer to maintain the pH at 7.4. This should be done at least 20 min before commencing the experiment.
5. Fill the compliance chamber (20 mL syringe) with 5 mL of buffer and 45 mL of air; this works to mimic the compliant walls of the aorta in vivo to allow for consistency in systolic and diastolic cycles and consistent perfusion.
6. Calibrate the pressure transducers following the manufacturer's instructions.
7. Fill both pressure transducers with ultrapure water, tighten caps, and ensure there are no air bubbles.
8. Ensure that all tubings are connected properly, and prime the perfusion system with oxygenated perfusion buffer, ensuring all air bubbles are eliminated.
9. Insert the polyethersulfone membrane, 0.45 μM filter above the bubble trap/heat chamber (*see* **Note 5**).
10. Place the cardioplegic solution on ice and gas with carbogen (95% O_2 and 5% CO_2) prior to excision of the heart.

3.2 Metal Cannula

1. Obtain a short metal 20-gauge needle.
2. Create two grooves, approximately 2–3 mm from the end of the needle for securing with suture (*see* **Note 6**).

3.3 Left Ventricular Balloon Catheter

3.3.1 LV Balloon Using Food Wrap

1. Obtain a blunted metal 20 gauge needle and attach the needle to a syringe filled with ultrapure water.
2. Attach a PE-100 polyethylene tube to the needle and ensure it is secure and leakproof.
3. Cut a circular piece of domestic cling film (saran wrap), about 25 mm in diameter.

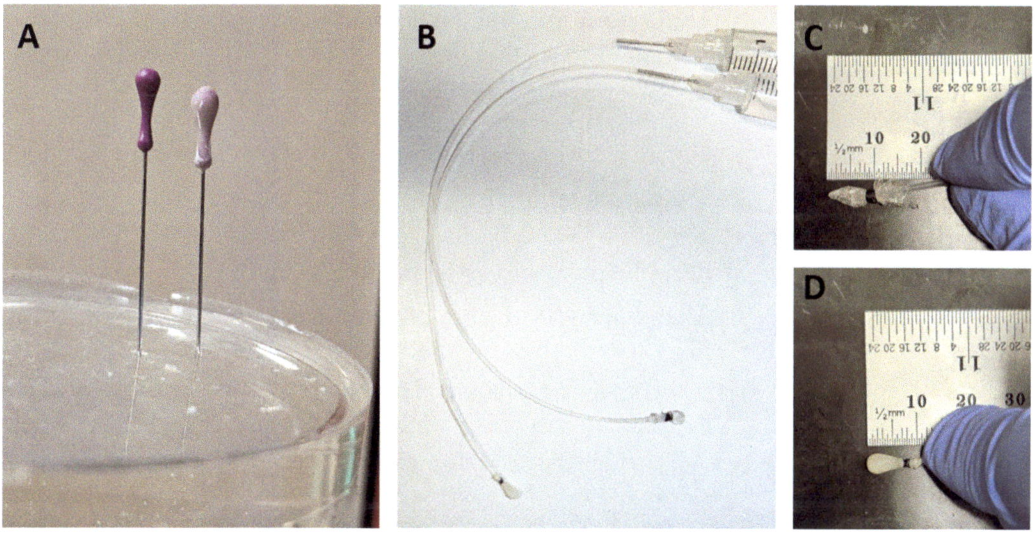

Fig. 2 Left ventricular balloon for measuring contractility. (**a**) Sewing pins, without latex and coated with latex. (**b**) Balloons made from latex and food wrap. (**c**) Partially deflated food wrap balloon. (**d**) Partially deflated latex balloon

4. Place the tubing slightly below the center of the cling film and wrap the cling film around the blunted polyethylene tube preferably with a blunted edge.
5. Fold the saran wrap over the end of the tube and leave a small space between the tube and the fold of the cling film.
6. Repeat the fold on the sides while gently turning the tube to make sure the cling wrap is wrapped around it until it achieves a spherical form.
7. Using your thumb and forefinger, ensure a tight seal of the cling wrap around the tube.
8. Tie the saran wrap to the tube using a 4–0 suture loosely at the base of the tube close to the cling wrap (*see* Fig. 2).
9. Inflate the balloon using the syringe, and ensure that there are no air bubbles which could dampen the pressure signal.
10. Tie the knot securely by continuously winding the thread, from the base of the balloon to slightly above the tube to form a single layer thread (*see* **Note 7**).
11. Inspect the balloon for air bubbles before tying a second suture to prevent any leaks.
12. Inflate the balloon to ensure it can accommodate 15–35 μL of water (*see* **Note 8**). Carefully detach the needle from the syringe making sure not to introduce any air bubbles.
13. Attach the balloon to the pressure transducer. When not in use, immerse and store in distilled water.

14. To control balloon volume, attach a pre-filled Hamilton 100 μL threaded plunger syringe to the side arm of the transducer.

3.3.2 LV Balloon Using Latex

1. Obtain a sewing pin with a large ball head measuring 3 mm.
2. Dip the pin head approximately 1 cm into liquid latex twice and allow to air dry for 3 h. When dry, it should appear clear.
3. Reapply the next layer by dipping again in latex.
4. After 2–3 layers of latex, place the balloons in a drying oven at 37 °C overnight.
5. To remove the balloons from the pin head, immerse in water for 2–3 h or rub gently while pulling apart, using baby powder.
6. Detach the balloons from the pin head, gently to prevent it from ripping.
7. Attach the latex balloon to a water-filled PE-50 and PE-100 tubing and attach to the pressure transducer.
8. When not in use, store the balloon in distilled water.

3.4 Heart Excision

1. Weigh the mouse (*see* **Note 9**).
2. Inject the mouse intraperitoneally with anticoagulant, heparin (1000 IU/kg), and wait for 15 min. The anticoagulation is to help prevent any blood clots in the excised heart.
3. Prepare the cannulation area. Turn on the microscope and light source.
4. Detach the cannula from the Langendorff rig and attach to a 1 mL syringe.
5. Place a petri dish containing ice-cold cardioplegic solution under the microscope.
6. Mount the syringe below the microscope with the cannula sitting in the petri dish.
7. Attach a suture loosely just above the grooves where the aorta will sit.
8. Induce anesthesia using isoflurane (5% at 0.5 L/min of oxygen) (*see* **Note 10**).
9. Confirm deep anesthesia by the loss of withdrawal response to toe pinch.
10. Commence thoracotomy. Pull up the mouse fur from the mid-abdomen by pinching and cutting with scissors.
11. Cut the diaphragm back bilaterally. Cut the rib cage on both sides, raise and clip back, to expose the thoracic cavity.

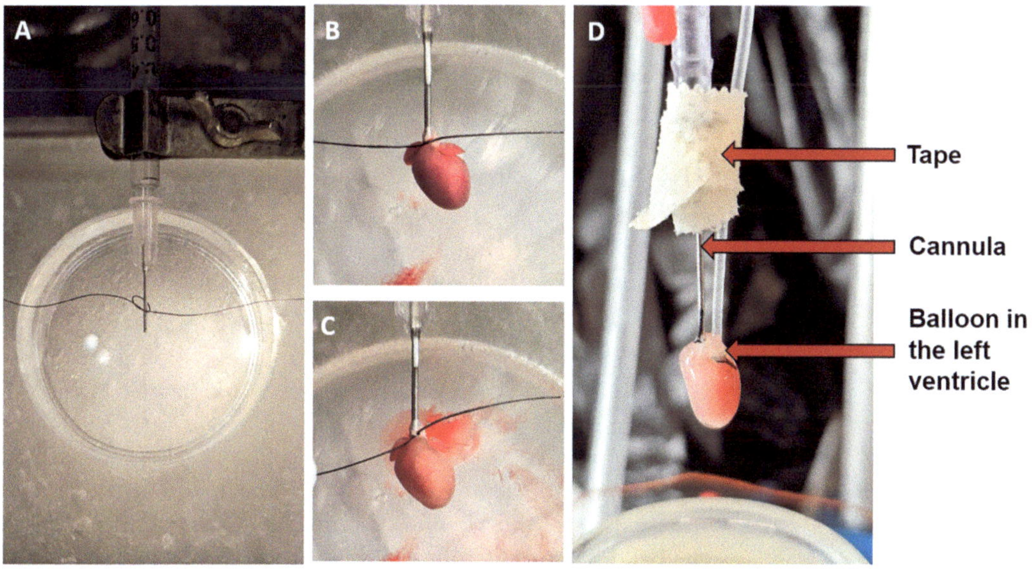

Fig. 3 Cannulation of the mouse heart. (**a**) Cannulation chamber with petri dish filled with cardioplegic solution, cannula (attached to a filled syringe) and 4–0 suture immersed in the ice-cold cardioplegic solution. (**b**) Ligated aorta on the cannula. (**c**) Perfusion buffer pushed through the heart to clear the blood. (**d**) Mouse heart hanging from a cannula with the balloon inserted into the left ventricle

12. Identify and gently remove the thymus to expose the aorta, and then clip the aorta, making sure to leave sufficient aortic length for cannulation without blocking coronary ostia.
13. Excise the heart and immediately place in a beaker containing the ice-cold cardioplegic solution to prevent any ischemic injury.
14. Transfer the heart to an ice-cold petri dish containing the same cardioplegic solution for cannulation (*see* **Note 11**).
15. While the heart is in the ice-cold solution, identify the aorta and move the heart close to the cannula (*see* **Note 12**).
16. Using two pairs of fine curved forceps, carefully grab both edges of the aorta and pull up like a sock on the cannula. If the aorta appears loose on the cannula, clamp the aorta with a small, blunted clip. Using a 4–0 silk suture, make a loose tie (*see* **Note 13**).
17. Slowly perfuse the heart with KHB. Correct cannulation is confirmed when the washout of blood from the epicardial coronary arteries is visualized. Proceed to make a knot with the suture (*see* Fig. 3).
18. Lift the heart on the cannula from the ice-cold solution and attach to the perfusion system. Ensure that the contractile function of the heart has restarted.
19. Trim away excess fat and tissue if required.

20. Start the recording on the acquisition system. Monitor the physiological parameters on the software interface. Once the coronary pressure of 80 mmHg is attained, hold the pressure to begin the constant pressure mode. Temperature should be approximately 37 °C in the tubing and 37.4 °C at the heart. This can be measured by placing a temperature probe close to the heart.
21. Allow the heart to equilibrate on the column for 5 min before insertion of the balloon. Normal rate for buffer through the mouse heart should be 1–5 mL/min.
22. Using an in-line flow probe, coronary flow should be monitored to ensure it stays within the acceptable range (*see* Table 1 and **Note 14**).

3.5 Insertion of LV Pressure Balloon

1. Open the stopcock connected to an open-ended syringe reserved to fill the Hamilton syringe and the balloon. Deflate the balloon, and carefully roll the balloon into a cone shape and turn the stopcock to ensure the balloon does not fill back up.
2. Identify the left atrium and using a small pair of scissors, carefully cut it off sufficient to expose the mitral (atrioventricular) valve.
3. Push the balloon gently and carefully into the left ventricle through the mitral valve.
4. Secure the balloon to the heart using a tape around the stopcock holding the cannula or tie the neck of the balloon the cannula using a suture. Ensure that this is firm to prevent the balloon from popping out if the heart develops strong contractions.
5. The pressure transducer should detect the contractility and reflect it as a change in pressure on the analysis software.
6. Open the stopcock and inflate the balloon gently with ~5 μL of water via the syringe to stretch the myocardial fibers until the end-diastolic pressure exceeds zero.
7. Continually increase the volume of fluid in the balloon at an increment of 2–5 μL until an end-diastolic pressure between 5 and 10 mmHg is achieved (*see* **Note 15**). Close the stopcock with each increment to maintain a closed system between the balloon and transducer. This allows the pressure transducer to detect the left ventricular pressure.
8. Lower the heart into the heated organ chamber filled with the perfusion buffer and cover the chamber (*see* **Note 16**).
9. Cover the organ chamber with paraffin or saran wrap.

3.6 Experimental Protocol

1. Allow the heart to stabilize for 20–30 min. Monitor the LV pressure trace for consistent steady-state pressure development and normal heart rhythm before obtaining basal heart function parameters.
2. Ensure that all parameters are being recorded including LV developed pressure (60–100 mmHg), coronary pressure (80 mmHg), coronary flow (1–5 mL/min), heart rate (>250 mmHg), and temperature (37–37.4 °C).
3. Record baseline measurement before any intervention or drug administration. Drug can be administered by adding to the perfusion buffer or by attaching a pump injection at the side arm close to the heart.
4. For experiments involving pacing, an electrode can be hooked on to the ventricle and the reference electrode attached to the cannula (*see* **Note 17**).
5. To record ECG, electrodes can be positioned on the left and right ventricles, with the reference electrode placed in the organ bath close to the heart.
6. Coronary effluent for biochemical analysis can be obtained by placing a graduated cylinder/beaker below the organ bath to collect the overflowing fluid.

3.7 Termination of Experiment

1. Stop recording and save the tracings for offline analysis.
2. Remove the heart from the organ chamber and release the hold on the coronary pressure.
3. Cut off the atrial tissue and remove the heart from the cannula.
4. Place the heart in a dish and cut into sections as required for biochemical or histological analysis.
5. Flash-freeze the heart tissues in liquid nitrogen and store at − 80 °C for further studies.

3.8 Offline Analysis

From the LV developed pressure, the LabChart 8 software can determine left ventricular developed pressure (LVDP), heart rate (HR), and maximum and minimum rate of developed pressure (+dP/dt and −dP/dt). LVDP is the change in peak systolic pressure minus end-diastolic pressure. Heart rate is the number of beats per minute, calculated from the systolic and diastolic cycle duration. The +dP/dt is the steepest slope during the upstroke of the LV pressure curve, indicating rate of contraction and −dP/dt is the steepest slope during the downstroke of the LV pressure curve, indicating rate of relaxation. Any time point from the trace can be selected and analyzed to obtain the average for each parameter (*see* Fig. 4).

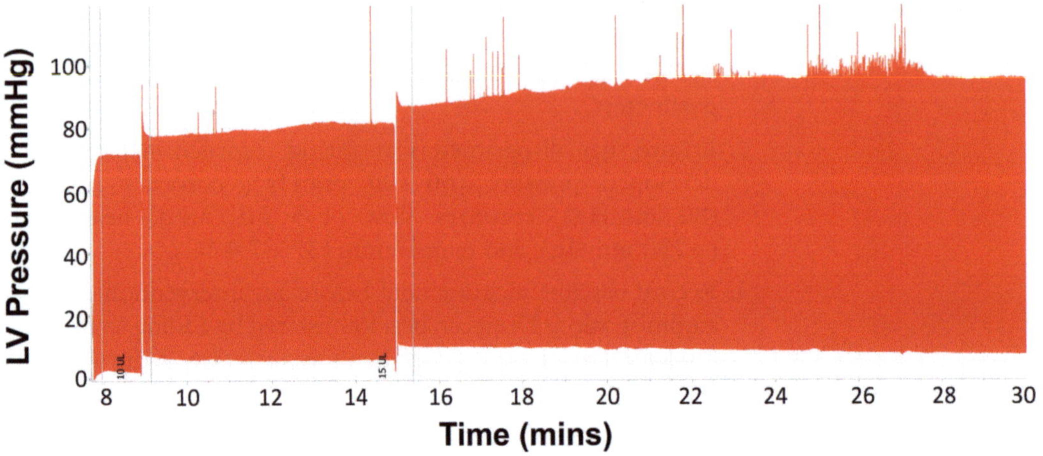

Fig. 4 A representative trace of LV developed pressure during the 30 min stabilization period, showing gradual increments in balloon volume and end-diastolic volume maintained between 5 and 10 mmHg

4 Notes

1. The Ca^{2+} concentration for experiments can vary depending on the experimental protocol. Typical concentrations used in different studies range from 1.35 to 2 mM. Glucose or other substrate levels can also be tuned for experimental aims.
2. Purchase or prepare stock solution of 1 M $CaCl_2$. Always add $CaCl_2$ to the Krebs–Henseleit buffer before use to prevent precipitation of Ca^{2+}. In addition, fresh buffer solutions can be made on the day or stock solutions without glucose and calcium can be prepared and stored in 4 °C.
3. A cardioplegic solution is used to arrest the heart. It contains high KCl and low $CaCl_2$. Approximately 100 mL of this solution is sufficient for dissection of one mouse heart.
4. To monitor the temperature of the heart, place a temperature probe/thermistor in the organ bath close to the heart. It is important to constantly monitor the temperature (36.5–37.4 °C) as this will affect the performance of the heart.
5. This helps to eliminate any air bubbles in the tubing closer to the heart.
6. The size of the needle depends on the rodent. For mouse, 20 G or 21 G needle would be suitable. A groove is made at the distal end of the cannula by engraving a rim around the distal end of the cannula. This groove is for the suture that secures the aorta to the cannula.

7. Ensure to create a single layer thread in order to reduce the bulkiness that may cause an irritation when the balloon is inserted through the mitral valve.
8. A high-volume balloon is not ideal as it may not fit into the heart. Measure the size of the balloon to contain about 25–30 μL of fluid for a mouse heart. The larger the animal heart, the larger the balloon size (for rats, 50–70 μL). To store the balloon, remove the plunger in the syringe, fill the syringe with water, and reattach to the balloon. It can be stored upright. It is also important to consider that the properties of the cling film will change over time. It is helpful to make many balloons and change frequently in between experiments.
9. Adequate care during animal handling should be taken to keep the animal from being stressed.
10. Alternative approved anesthesia methods can be used instead of the inhalation of volatile agents such as isoflurane (as we do).
11. The total duration from when ventilation stops or when the chest is opened (if the mouse is being ventilated) to cannulation and reperfusion, must be kept under 3 min to prevent damage or ischemic preconditioning and ensure viable heart function.
12. There are two methods for cannulation. The cannulation can be done in a petri dish with the cannula attached to a syringe filled with KH buffer. After cannulation, the cannula with the excised heart is detached from the syringe and attached to the perfusion system. The other method is to directly hang the heart on the cannula while it is still attached to the perfusion system. This second method works better for larger hearts.
13. Extra care should be taken while inserting the cannula. The cannula should not be inserted too far into the aorta, and this would cause an occlusion of the ostia of the left and right coronary arteries. Normally, on a 20-gauge syringe needle, the aorta should stay on and not fall off. However, you can still secure the aorta with a clip.
14. Coronary flow can be measured in real time using an in-line flow probe in the perfusion line. Coronary flow can also be determined from the pressure pump controller used to maintain constant perfusion pressure. High coronary flow could be an indication of a tear in the aorta, and low coronary flow may indicate that there is an air bubble in the coronary circulation therefore inadequate perfusion.
15. Make small increments of 2–5 μL while observing the change in end-diastolic pressure and LV developed pressure. High fluid volume in the balloon can lead to tissue compression and could trigger arrhythmias; therefore, an excessively high volume should be avoided.

16. Fill the chamber with buffer just before the heart is lowered into the organ bath.
17. For pacing, a bipolar stimulator is recommended to prevent toxicity because of electrolysis of the perfusion fluid.

References

1. Bell RM, Mocanu MM, Yellon DM (2011) Retrograde heart perfusion: the Langendorff technique of isolated heart perfusion. J Mol Cell Cardiol 50(6):940–950
2. Sutherland FJ, Hearse DJ (2000) The isolated blood and perfusion fluid perfused heart. Pharmacol Res 41(6):613–627
3. Hearse DJ, Sutherland FJ (2000) Experimental models for the study of cardiovascular function and disease. Pharmacol Res 41(6):597–603
4. Langendorff O (1895) Untersuchungen am überlebenden Säugethierherzen. Archiv für die gesamte Physiologie des Menschen und der Tiere 61(6):291–332
5. Skrzypiec-Spring M, Grotthus B, Szeląg A, Schulz R (2007) Isolated heart perfusion according to Langendorff—still viable in the new millennium. J Pharmacol Toxicol Methods 55(2):113–126
6. Liao R, Podesser BK, Lim CC (2012) The continuing evolution of the Langendorff and ejecting murine heart: new advances in cardiac phenotyping. Am J Phys Heart Circ Phys 303(2):H156–H167
7. Reichelt ME, Willems L, Hack BA, Peart JN, Headrick JP (2009) Cardiac and coronary function in the Langendorff-perfused mouse heart model. Exp Physiol 94(1):54–70
8. Curtis M, Macleod B, Tabrizchi R, Walker M (1986) An improved perfusion apparatus for small animal hearts. J Pharmacol Methods 15(1):87–94
9. Sutherland FJ, Shattock MJ, Baker KE, Hearse DJ (2003) Mouse isolated perfused heart: characteristics and cautions. Clin Exp Pharmacol Physiol 30(11):867–878
10. Miller A, Wright GL (2011) Fabrication of murine ventricular balloons for the langendorff heart preparation. J Biotechnol Biomater 1: 101
11. Sumeray MS, Yellon DM (1998) Characterisation and validation of a murine model of global ischaemia-reperfusion injury. Mol Cell Biochem 186:61–68
12. Headrick JP, Peart J, Hack B, Flood A, Matherne GP (2001) Functional properties and responses to ischaemia-reperfusion in Langendorff perfused mouse heart. Exp Physiol 86(6):703–716

Chapter 10

Exosome Isolation from Pericardial Fluids

Dhananjie N. K. Chandrasekera

Abstract

Extracellular vehicles such as exosomes which lie in the size range of 30–150 nm have gained significant attention due to their ability to contain molecular cargoes. These vesicles are released by various cells and are found to stably carry their molecular cargoes to recipient cells via different biological fluids. Therefore, exosomes isolated from various fluids such as plasma, urine, and pericardial fluid have been extensively studied in recent years. However, due to the miniscule nature of exosomes, isolation of exosomes from biological fluids has been a challenge, mainly due to low yields, contamination from large vesicles and proteins, and variable starting sample volumes. The following protocol describes the isolation of exosomes from human pericardial fluid samples collected from patients undergoing coronary artery bypass graft surgery. The exosomes isolated from these samples have been previously shown to have increased expression of cardiovascular molecular markers. Due to the precious nature of the patient samples, the exosomes isolated from this protocol have been validated to confirm their purity and viability for downstream applications.

Key words Extracellular vesicles, Exosomes, Nanovesicles, Precipitation, Size exclusion chromatography, Pericardial fluid

1 Introduction

Exosomes are a class of extracellular vesicles that lie within the 30–150 nm size range. These vesicles are released by various cells and are stable in various types of biological fluids. Research into exosomes has increased in recent years owing to the functional and biomarker capabilities of exosomes [1–3]. Prior to exosome release by host cells, various types of RNAs, enzymes, and proteins are shuttled into immature exosomes during their biogenesis [3]. Once released by their host cells, exosomes can be found to be stable in various extracellular or biological fluids [3–6]. Furthermore, due to the miniscule nature of the exosomes, as well as the surface markers that they express, these exosomes are easily taken up by recipient cells to have various functional effects [3–5, 7, 8]. These

Dhananjie N. K. Chandrasekera and Rajesh Katare (eds.), *Cardiomyocytes: Methods and Protocols*, Methods in Molecular Biology, vol. 2894, https://doi.org/10.1007/978-1-0716-4342-6_10,

characteristics make exosomes a promising avenue for therapeutic and biomarker research.

Since their discovery, the methods in which exosomes have been isolated have been under development [1, 9–12]. In fact, exosomes can now be isolated from various biological fluids, such as plasma, saliva, urine, and pericardial fluid [4–9, 11, 12]. Most studies have optimized the isolation of exosomes from biological fluids, such as plasma and urine, with high volumes and abundance [3, 5, 11]. Isolation of exosomes from low-volume and abundant biological fluids, such as pericardial fluid samples, requires extra attention because of their precious nature [4, 12]. Early isolation protocols use a series of large g forces to pellet exosomes; however, these isolation protocols have the potential to compromise the exosomal structure as well as result in impure exosome isolations [1, 13–15]. Therefore, considering the downstream applications of the isolated exosomes, the process by which exosomes are isolated should result in high-quality exosomes with high quantities and purity.

The exosome isolation protocol detailed in this chapter utilizes a combination of reagent-based exosome precipitation and size exclusion chromatography (SEC). Individually, exosomes isolated by precipitation or SEC result in final exosome isolation of varying quality. However, when combined, the following protocol consistently yielded pure exosomes in high abundance.

2 Materials

1. Precipitation-based exosome isolation reagent (*see* **Note 1**).
2. Size exclusion chromatography (SEC)-based exosome isolation columns (*see* **Note 2**).
3. Stand to hold exosome isolation columns vertically.
4. 2 mL Eppendorf tubes.
5. Amicon centrifugal tubes, 10 kDa capacity, 15 mL.
6. 0.2 μm syringe filters.
7. 1 mL syringes.
8. 0.2 μm vacuum filters.
9. Centrifuge capable of cooling up to 4 °C and speeds up to 10,000× *g*.
10. Phosphate-buffered saline (PBS): NaCl 137 mM, KCl 2.7 mM, Na_2HPO_4 10 mM, KH_2PO_4 1.8 mM, pH 7.4 (*see* **Note 3**).
11. Sodium azide (0.05% w/v in PBS) (*see* **Note 3**).
12. Sodium hydroxide solution 0.5 M (*see* **Note 3**).

3 Methods

3.1 Sample Preparation: Samples Can Be Either Fresh from Surgery or Frozen

1. On receiving samples from the operating theatre, centrifuge the samples at 250× *g* for 15 min at 4 °C.
2. Collect the supernatant, avoiding any large tissue debris that come through during sample collection (*see* **Note 4**).
3. Filter the sample though a 0.2 μm syringe filter using a 1 mL syringe to remove cellular debris.
4. The filtered sample is now ready for exosome precipitation.

3.2 Exosome Precipitation

1. Mix the sample with the precipitation reagent in a 1:1 ratio in an appropriately sized Eppendorf tube (*see* **Note 5**).
2. Mix the sample and reagent solution using either a pipette or vortex, until the mixture is a homogenous solution.
3. Incubate the mixture at 4 °C or ice for 1 h (*see* **Note 6**).
4. Centrifuge the mixture at 10,000× *g* for 1 h at 4 °C.
5. Remove the supernatant without disturbing the pellet containing exosomes (*see* **Note 7**).
6. Gently resuspend the pellet in filtered PBS to a final volume of 500 μL (*see* **Notes 8** and **9**).
7. The vesicle suspension is now ready for exosome purification.

3.3 Exosome Purification

1. Set up the SEC column vertically, with the loading frit at the top, on its stand and let in equilibrate to room temperature (*see* **Note 10**).
2. Label the Eppendorf tubes that will be used for the collection of the flow through of the columns, based on the volume fraction that will be collected (*see* **Note 11**).
3. Gently remove the stop-caps on either side of the column, without damaging the resin of the column.
4. Wash the column with 1.5× the column volume (volume of buffer required to fill the column) of PBS. Allow the buffer to wash through the column before any sample is added into the loading frit at the top of the column.
5. Add 500 μL of the vesicle suspension into the loading frit of the column. Collect the flow through at the bottom of the column as the vesicle suspension flows though the column. The flow through should be collected in the form of 500 μL fractions. The flow through collected from additions of the vesicle suspension will be the first fraction.
6. Once the vesicle suspension has flown into the column, the flow through from the bottom of the column will stop. Users should wait till the suspension is completely in the column

before adding in any buffers for exosome purification (*see* **Note 12**).

7. Add the PBS in increments of 500 μL at a time. Allow the PBS to fully flow into the column before adding the next volume of PBS. This should be done a total of nine times, thereby resulting in nine more fractions.
8. Fractions 1–6 should be kept aside as they would consist of the buffer volume of the column as well as non-exosome contaminants (*see* **Note 12**).
9. Fractions 7–10 should be collected and immediately stored on ice as they would contain the exosome-containing fractions (*see* **Note 12**).
10. Concentrate the seventh, eighth, ninth, and tenth fractions by adding them into the filtration insert of the Amicon-Ultra 4 centrifugation filter. Centrifuge the fractions at 7000× *g* for 45 min at 4 °C.
11. Concentrated purified exosomes will be at the bottom of the filtration insert. Depending on the number of exosomes in the sample, approximately 50–100 μL of buffer will be remaining.
12. Pipette the concentrated exosomes in the filtration insert a few times to ensure an even suspension.
13. Transfer the exosomes into a new labeled tube. The exosome sample can be used for downstream applications or stored at −80 °C for later use (*see* **Note 13**).
14. If another sample is to be purified using the same column, the column should be flushed with 1× buffer volume of sodium hydroxide solution and 3× buffer volume of PBS. If sample collection is complete, and the column is to be stored, it should have a wash with the sodium azide buffer.

4 Notes

1. This reagent is used to precipitate the exosomes in the pericardial fluid samples to separate them from the majority of the proteins and large vesicles. However, by itself, the reagent results in aggregated clumps of vesicles as well as contamination with non-exosomal large vesicles. Therefore, this protocol uses a secondary purification step using size exclusion chromatography.
2. Based on each individual experiment/study needs, the type of exosome isolation column that is used can be changed. For the purpose of this protocol, exosomes were isolated from human pericardial fluid samples using QEVOriginal (30 nm) SEC columns from Izon. As per the need of the user, columns

from alternate manufacturers can be used, with prior assessment of the compatibility of the product with the requirements of this protocol. The columns must be equilibrated according to manufacturer's instructions prior to exosome isolation.

3. All buffers must be equilibrated to room temperature and filtered through either a 0.2 μm syringe filter or vacuum filter.
4. Samples can be stored in −80 °C after this step in appropriately labeled Eppendorf tubes. When preparing for exosome isolation, frozen samples should be thawed on ice.
5. The ratio of sample to precipitation reagent would vary depending on the reagent specifications. Refer to manufacturer instructions to determine the optimal ratio most suitable for exosome precipitation.
6. The sample/reagent mixture can be incubated for a longer period depending on time constraints. However, users should refer to the manufacturer protocol to determine the optimal timeframe most suitable for exosome precipitation based on the reagent used.
7. Depending on the amount of starting sample volume, and the amount of exosomes available in the starting sample, the pellet may or may not be visible. Therefore, it is best practice to orientate all tubes in the centrifuge so that the pellet would collect at a specific part of the tube during centrifugation.
8. If the pellet is larger and sticky, store the resuspended pellet at 4 °C for 1–2 h. The pellet should slowly start to dissolve into the PBS. Gently pipette the solution a few times to ensure a homogenous vesicle suspension.
9. The vesicle suspension can be stored at −80 °C after this step in appropriately labeled Eppendorf tubes for exosome purification later. If so, the sample should be thawed at 4° or on ice before purification. The sample should be visually inspected to ensure that there are no aggregates, undissolved pellet, or ice prior to exosome purification using SEC.
10. Prior to exosome purification, the columns should be visually inspected to ensure that there are not any cracks, bubbles, or salt buildup in the columns (especially if a reusable column has been taken out of storage after a previous use). Columns with compromised resin integrity will significantly affect the quality and the purity of the final exosome sample.
11. The volume of flow through and the collected fraction numbers may vary depending on the columns that are being used. Therefore, it is best to refer to the manufacturer protocol to determine the fractions and volumes that need to be collected by the user.

12. Users must wait till the suspension has completely flown into the column before adding in any buffers for exosome purification. The addition of buffers to the loading frit allows for the suspension to flow through the SEC column. As the suspension flows though, the contents within it will be separated according to their sizes. Therefore, the resulting flow through fractions will have various particles/vesicles/proteins based on their size. Depending on the type of column used, the optimal exosome-containing fractions would vary. Therefore, users must refer to the manufacturer protocol or carry out optimization trials to determine the optimal exosome-containing fractions. For this protocol, fractions 1–6 (according to manufacturer protocols) had no exosomes, while fractions 7–10 were exosome-containing fractions.
13. Exosomes isolated using this protocol have been validated by the author to confirm their quantity and purity using western blotting, transmission electron microscopy, immuno-gold labeling, and dynamic light scattering. The user should also validate the quality of the exosomes isolated by themselves to ensure that the protocol provides exosomes that are suitable for their experimental needs.

Acknowledgements

The research detailed in this chapter was supported by a Smart Idea Project Grant "Cell free approach for the treatment of ischemic diabetic ulcer" (UOOX2205) from the Ministry of Business, Innovation and Employment to Assosc. Prof. Rajesh Katare (R.K.), Explorer Research Grant from the Health Research Council, NZ (22/632) to R.K., and the PhD consumables fund from the Department of Physiology, University of Otago. D.N.K.C was supported by the University of Otago Doctoral Scholarship. D.N.K.C is now affiliated with the Department of Cardiac Physiology, National Cerebral and Cardiovascular Center, Osaka, Japan.

References

1. Dvorak HF, Quay SC, Orenstein NS, Dvorak AM, Hahn P, Bitzer AM, Carvalho AC (1981) Tumor shedding and coagulation. Science 212(4497):923–924
2. Pan BT, Teng K, Wu C, Adam M, Johnstone RM (1985) Electron microscopic evidence for externalization of the transferrin receptor in vesicular form in sheep reticulocytes. J Cell Biol 101(3):942–948
3. Chandrasekera D, Katare R (2022) Exosomal microRNAs in diabetic heart disease. Cardiovasc Diabetol 21(1):122
4. Beltrami C, Besnier M, Shantikumar S, Shearn AI, Rajakaruna C, Laftah A et al (2017) Human pericardial fluid contains exosomes enriched with cardiovascular-expressed microRNAs and promotes therapeutic angiogenesis. Mol Ther 25(3):679–693
5. Emanueli C, Shearn AI, Laftah A, Fiorentino F, Reeves BC, Beltrami C et al (2016) Coronary

artery-bypass-graft surgery increases the plasma concentration of exosomes carrying a cargo of cardiac microRNAs: an example of exosome trafficking out of the human heart with potential for cardiac biomarker discovery. PLoS One 11(4):e0154274

6. Keller S, Rupp C, Stoeck A, Runz S, Fogel M, Lugert S et al (2007) CD24 is a marker of exosomes secreted into urine and amniotic fluid. Kidney Int 72(9):1095–1102
7. Tian T, Wang Y, Wang H, Zhu Z, Xiao Z (2010) Visualizing of the cellular uptake and intracellular trafficking of exosomes by live-cell microscopy. J Cell Biochem 111(2):488–496
8. Salomon C, Scholz-Romero K, Sarker S, Sweeney E, Kobayashi M, Correa P et al (2016) Gestational diabetes mellitus is associated with changes in the concentration and bioactivity of placenta-derived exosomes in maternal circulation across gestation. Diabetes 65(3):598–609
9. Martins TS, Catita J, Rosa IM, da Cruz e Silva OAB, Henriques AG (2018) Exosome isolation from distinct biofluids using precipitation and column-based approaches. PLoS One 13: e0198820. https://doi.org/10.1371/journal.pone.0198820
10. Théry C, Amigorena S, Raposo G, Clayton A (2006) Isolation and characterization of exosomes from cell culture supernatants and biological fluids. Chapter 3, unit 22. In: Bonifacino JS, Dasso M, Harford JB, Lippincott-Schwartz J, Yamada KM (eds) Current protocols in cell biology. Wiley, Hoboken, pp 1–29
11. Shtam T, Evtushenko V, Samsonov R, Zabrodskaya Y, Kamyshinsky R, Zabegina L et al (2020) Evaluation of immune and chemical precipitation methods for plasma exosome isolation. PLoS One 15(11):e0242732
12. Chandrasekera D, Shah R, van Hout I, De Jonge W, Bunton R, Parry D et al (2023) Combination of precipitation and size exclusion chromatography as an effective method for exosome like extracellular vesicle isolation from pericardial fluids. Nano 7(4):345
13. Skottvoll FYS, Berg HE, BjØrseth K, Lund K, Roos N, Bekhradnia S et al (2019) Ultracentrifugation versus kit exosome isolation: nanoLC–MS and other tools reveal similar performance biomarkers, but also contaminations. Future Sci OA 5(1):FSO359
14. Baranyai T, Herczeg K, Onódi Z, Voszka I, Módos K, Marton N et al (2015) Isolation of exosomes from blood plasma: qualitative and quantitative comparison of ultracentrifugation and size exclusion chromatography methods. PLoS One 10(12):e0145686
15. Dash M, Palaniyandi K, Ramalingam S, Sahabudeen S, Raja NS (2021) Exosomes isolated from two different cell lines using three different isolation techniques show variation in physical and molecular characteristics. Biochim Biophys Acta Biomembr 1863(2): 183490

Chapter 11

Quantitative Real-Time PCR for Circular RNA Detection and Analysis

Amit Kumar Rai and Venkata Naga Srikanth Garikipati

Abstract

In eukaryotes, nearly 2% of the genome represented by the coding proteins. However, emerging evidence suggest more than 75% of the human genome referred to as noncoding part also plays a crucial role in governing major regulatory pathways. Noncoding RNAs can be categorized into several groups, such as microRNAs (miRNAs), small nuclear RNA (snRNAs), small nucleolar RNA (snoRNAs), transfer RNA (tRNA), and circular RNA (circRNAs), which contribute to this regulatory landscape. Circular RNAs (circRNAs) are identified as a new class of regulatory noncoding RNAs with gene regulatory roles by acting as miRNA or RNA binding protein sponges or interacting with proteins. Researchers employ quantitative real-time PCR methods to examine circular RNA expression utilizing divergent primers for identification and quantification.

Key words Circular RNA, RNase R, q-RT PCR, Divergent primer

1 Introduction

Circular RNAs (circRNAs) have emerged as a novel class of regulatory noncoding RNAs exhibiting gene regulatory roles by acting as miRNA or RNA binding protein sponges or interacting with proteins [1–3]. Circular RNAs result from back-splicing events, forming covalently closed circular RNA molecules [2, 4]. Advanced deep RNA sequencing techniques unveiled tissue-specific expression pattern of circular RNAs in various eukaryotes [5, 6]. CircRNAs have been implicated in various diseases including cancer, diabetes, heart diseases, and neurodegenerative disorders [1, 7–9]. Circular RNAs are increasingly recognized as potential candidates as disease biomarkers, therapeutic targets, and vaccine candidates [10–12]. Despite their significance, validating circRNA expression typically relies on quantitative real-time polymerase chain reaction (qRT-PCR). This protocol provides essential steps for characterizing circRNA expression from a given tissue or cell.

Dhananjie N. K. Chandrasekera and Rajesh Katare (eds.), *Cardiomyocytes: Methods and Protocols*, Methods in Molecular Biology, vol. 2894, https://doi.org/10.1007/978-1-0716-4342-6_11,

2 Materials

We outline the steps required for the detection of a specific circular RNA in tissues and cells after RNA sequencing.

2.1 RNA Isolation and Quantification

- miRNeasy tissue/cells advanced micro kit (Cat # 217684, Qiagen, USA).
- Ethanol for molecular biology (Cat # 108543, Millipore-Sigma, USA).
- Isopropanol for molecular biology (Cat # I9516, Millipore-Sigma, USA).
- 4 °C microcentrifuge (Cat # 5418R, Eppendorf, USA).
- Mini vortexer (Cat # 58816-121, VWR Scientific, USA).
- Accu-jet pro pipette (Cat # 19 M94220, Accu-jet, Germany).
- NanoDrop One spectrophotometer (Cat # ND-ONE-W, Thermo Fisher Scientific, USA).
- RNase R (Epicenter Technologies, Madison, WI).
- Nuclease-free tips including 10 μL, 20–200 μL, 1000 μL (Genesee Scientific, USA).
- Ultrapure nuclease-free water (Cat # 10977015, Invitrogen, USA) .
- PureLink RNA mini kit (Cat # 12183018A, Invitrogen, USA).

2.2 c-DNA Preparation and Real-Time PCR

- High-capacity c-DNA reverse transcription kit (Cat # 4374966, Applied Biosystems, USA).
- Power Up SYBR green master mix (Cat # A25741, Applied Biosystems, USA).
- Mini Amp Thermal Cycler (Cat # A37834, Applied Biosystems, USA).
- QuantStudio real-time PCR system (QuantStudio 3.0, Applied Biosystems, USA).
- MicroAmp Fast 96-well reaction plate (0.1 mL) (Cat # 4346907, Applied Biosystems, USA).
- MicroAmp optical adhesive film (Cat # 4360954, Applied Biosystems, USA).
- Filter pipette tips (nuclease-free, 10 μL, 20–200 μL, 1000 μL—Genessee, USA).
- Microcentrifuge tube (0.5 mL, 1.5 mL, 2.0 mL nuclease-free, Genessee, USA).
- PlateFuge™ Microplate Microcentrifuge with rotor and plate carrier (Cat # Z742569, PlateFuge).

3 Methods

In this protocol, all necessary steps will be carried out at room temperature unless otherwise specified.

3.1 Primer Designing

After RNA sequencing, we selected a specific circRNA or set of circRNAs to evaluate their expression under the given experimental conditions. To test the expression of circular RNA, we designed divergent primers (Fig. 1). Circular RNAs are covalently closed single-stranded RNA molecules that originate from back-splicing events (Kristensen et al., 2019), and they lack 5′ or 3′ ends. We will follow these steps to design primer:

1. First, mature sequences were obtained from circAtlas 3.0 [13].
2. Create a back-splicing junction (BSJ) by joining the 5′ and 3′ ends by counting 100 nucleotides on each side [14, 15].
3. Primers were designed using the BSJ sequence as a template (Fig. 1) using Primer 3 plus (https://www.primer3plus.com/index.html) or CIRCprimerXL [16].
4. Primers generated using this method were used to examine the expression of the desired circRNAs.

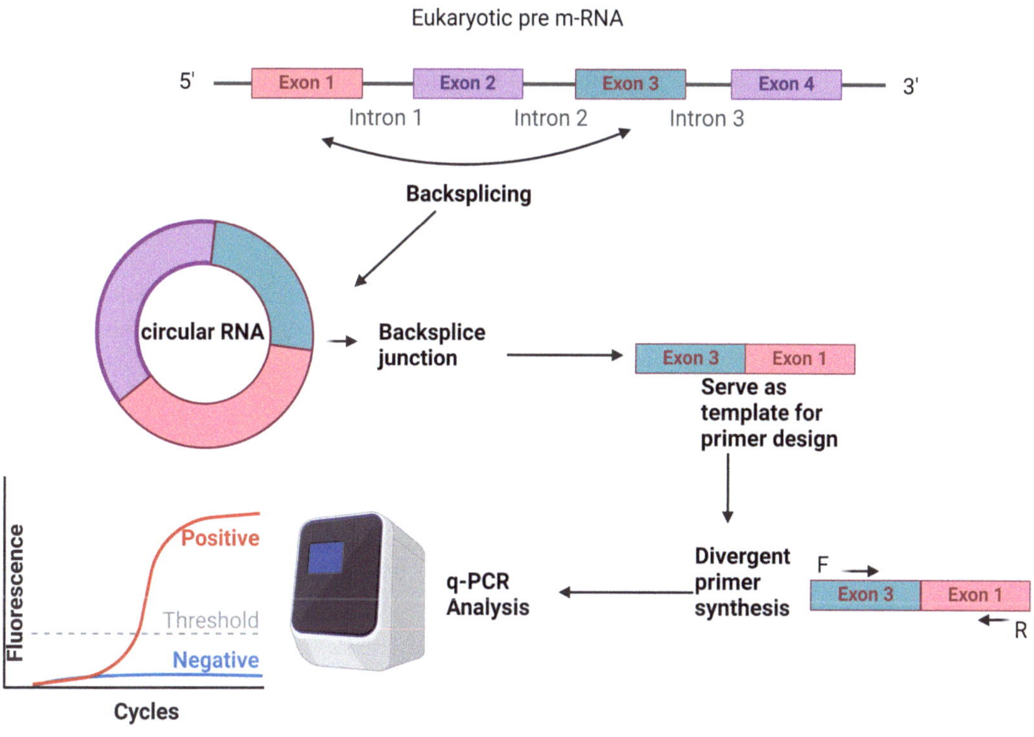

Fig. 1 Schematic outline of primer designing and characterization of circular RNA by quantitative real-time polymerase chain reaction (qRT-PCR)

3.2 RNA Isolation

1. RNA was isolated according to the manufacturer's protocol (miRNeasy kit, Cat # 217684, Qiagen, USA). This kit can be used for animal cells and tissues.
2. In brief, all buffers were equilibrated at room temperature before use.
3. Add an appropriate amount of ethanol to dissolve the RWT and RPE buffers (according to the manufacturer's protocol).
4. Approximately 260 μL of RLT buffer (provided by the manufacturer) was required for the homogenization of 0.5 million cells or 0.5 mg tissue.
5. Next, 40 μL of buffer AL (provided in the kit) was added and mixed thoroughly. The samples were maintained at room temperature for 3 min.
6. Transfer the lysates (cells/tissues lysed in RLT buffer + AL buffer) into a g-DNA eliminator column (provided with kit) in a 2.0 mL collection tube and centrifuge at ≥8000× *g* (≥10,000 *rpm*) for 30 s. The flow-through was kept for further steps, and the column was discarded.
7. While using tissue for RNA isolation, the flow-through was transferred from the previous step into a fresh 2.0 mL tube, and 20 μL of RPP buffer (provided with the kit) was immediately added. The mixture was then thoroughly vortexed for 20 s. Keep this tube at room temperature for 3 min (*see* **Note 1**).
8. After incubation for 3 min at room temperature, the pellet was centrifuged for 3 min at 12,000× *g* to precipitate the pellet (*see* **Note 1**).
9. Attention: After this step, the supernatant will be colorless and transparent. This supernatant was transferred to a fresh 2.0 mL tube (*see* **Note 2**).
10. Based on the volume of the supernatant, add 1.3 times of isopropanol, and titrate it. Now, transfer the supernatant + isopropanol solution to UCP column (provided with the kit) with 2.0 mL tube. Centrifuge it for 15 s at ≥8000 × *g*. Discard the flow-through and keep the column intact (*see* **Note 3**).
11. Next, add 700 μL of RWT buffer (make sure you added the required amount of ethanol into stock buffers as per manufacturer recommendations) in UCP column. Centrifuge it for 15 s at ≥8000× *g*. Discard the flow-through and keep the column intact.
12. Add 500 μL of RPE buffer (make sure you added the required amount of ethanol into the stock buffers as per manufacturer recommendations) in UCP column. Centrifuge it for 15 s at ≥8000× *g*. Discard the flow-through and keep the column intact.

13. Add 500 μL of ethanol (80%) into the UCP column and centrifuge it for 2 min at ≥8000× *g*. Discard the flow-through and collection tube (*see* **Note 4**).
14. The UCP mini column needs to dry as per manufacturer's instruction.
15. The UCP mini column is then placed in a new collection tube (1.5 mL provided in kit) for RNA elution. Add 20–30 μL of nuclease-free water to UCP column and incubate it for 1 min at room temperature. After 1 min of incubation, place this column with 1.5 mL tube in centrifuge and spin it at maximum speed for 1 min. Flow-through will be used to quantify RNA. Please avoid multiple freeze–thaw cycles of RNA to maintain the integrity of the samples (*see* **Note 5**).
16. RNA can be quantified immediately after elution or can be stored in freezer.
17. Eluted RNA can be treated with RNase R to avoid any linear RNA by adding 1 μL of 2.5 U of RNase R in 2 μL of 10× RNase R buffer, 1 μL of RNase R, and 0.5 μL of RiboLock, and adjust the volume with nuclease-free water in total 2.0–5.0 μg of RNA at 37 °C for 30 min (*see* **Note 6**).
18. Using RNA purification kit (Cat # 12183018A), purify control or RNase R-treated RNA and elute them in 20 μL of nuclease-free water.

3.3 c-DNA Synthesis

1. After quantification of RNA from the above step, 1 μg of RNA (control or RNase R-treated samples) will be used for c-DNA synthesis as per manufacturer recommendation (high-capacity cDNA reverse transcription kit, cat # 4374966, Applied Biosystems, USA).
2. This kit can be used to synthesize c-DNA using 1 μg of total RNA in a 20 μL of reaction.
3. Prepare a 2× reverse transcription reaction mixture for preparation of c-DNA.
4. Thaw every component of c-DNA synthesis kit on ice.
5. Prepare a 10 μL (Solution A) reaction by using RNA as per your desired amount (*see* **Note 7**).
6. Next, prepare a 10 μL (Solution B) of 2× reverse transcription mixture by adding following components as per Table 1 (*see* **Note 7**).
7. Then mix Solutions A and B to reach up to 20 μL of reaction volume (*see* **Note 7**).
8. This reaction mixture will be given a brief spin to mix it thoroughly (*see* **Note 8**).

Table 1
Various components and amounts needed for making a 20 μL reaction mixture for c-DNA synthesis

Components	Amount (per 20 μL reaction mixture)
10× RT-buffer	2.0 μL
25× dNTP	0.8 μL
10× random primer	2.0 μL
MultiScribe reverse transcriptase enzyme	1.0 μL
RNase inhibitor	1.0 μL
Nuclease-free water	3.2 μL
Total	**10.0 μL**

Table 2
An outlined setting of temperature and time for c-DNA synthesis

Setting	Step 1	Step 2	Step 3	Step 4
Temperature	25 °C	37 °C	85 °C	4 °C
Time	10 min	2 h	5 min	Hold

9. Proceed to set up for c-DNA synthesis as per suggestion of manufacturer's protocol (detailed in Table 2).
10. Set the reaction volume to 20 μL.
11. Now, load the samples in the thermal cycler and close the lid.
12. Run the software.
13. After around 2 h and 15 min, the sample will be ready to run for q-PCR.

3.4 Detection of circRNA by Q-RT PCR

1. Use synthesized c-DNA a template for qPCR from Subheading 3.3.
2. Primers synthesized from Subheading 3.2 will be used for setting q-PCR reaction.
   - Primers can be obtained from any manufacturer (e.g., IDT or Thermo Fisher Scientific) by providing them the sequences.
   - Primer sets can be chosen based on the chemistry of dye such as SYBR green or TaqMan.
   - For example: Power Up SYBR green master mix (Cat # A25741, Applied Biosystems, USA) is suitable for 1–10 ng of c-DNA (*see* **Note 9**).

Table 3
Components of q-RT PCR setup (based on SYBR Green chemistry)

Component	Volume (10 μL/well)	Volume (20 μL/well)
Power up SYBR master mix (2×)	5.0 μL	10 μL
Forward primer and reverse primer	1×[a] or 0.5–1.0 μM	1×[a] or 0.5–1.0 μM
Template c-DNA	1 ng–10 ng	1 ng–10 ng
Nuclease-free water	Till final volume is 10 μL	Till final volume is 20 μL
Total	**10.0 μL**	**20.0 μL**

[a]If primer was ordered by using the pre-dissolved primers of IDT

Table 4
An outlined setting of q-RT PCR in QuantStudio 3.0

Step	Temperature (°C)	Time	Cycle
UDG activation	50	2 min	1
Activation	95	2 min	1
Denaturation	95	1 s (for fast q-RT PCR) or 30 s (for standard q-RT PCR)	40
Annealing/ extension	60	30 s (for fast q-RT PCR) or 1 min (for standard q-RT PCR)	

3. User can set up reactions as per requirement based on the manufacturer's protocol.
   - An example experimental setup is indicated in Table 3.
4. Then add every reaction in 96-well PCR plates as per triplicate or tetraplicate.
5. Seal the 96-well plate with the help of an optical adhesive PCR plate sealer.
6. Give a brief spin in PCR plate microfuge to mix every component of Table 3 that is in the reaction mix.
7. Set up the reaction in QuantStudio 3.0 as per guidelines of the manufacturer (Table 4).
8. Load the PCR plate in machine and run the software (*see* **Note 10**).
9. Attention: Please make sure you have a right plate based on the block available in QuantStudio (e.g., if you are using 0.1 mL block in QuantStudio, then your plate should be compatible to the block).

3.5 Analysis of q-PCR Data

1. After retrieving the Ct from QuantStudio 3.0 software, one can utilize the quantification method by using $2^{e\ (\text{delta-Ct})}$.
2. 18 s r-RNA primer can be used as a loading control gene.

4 Notes

1. For cell culture, this step may be skipped.
2. You may also use 1.5 mL tube, depending upon the volume.
3. Any remaining sample can be repeated as above by using the same column.
4. It is important to prepare it in nuclease-free water.
5. From this step, RNA can be placed at ice or 4 °C until quantification and cDNA preparation. Otherwise, store RNA at −80 °C freezer for long-term storage.
6. Please keep one reaction without adding RNase R and it will serve as negative control.
7. Keep on ice.
8. Please do not vortex.
9. This kit is not recommended to set up a reaction mixture less than 10 μL.
10. In QuantStudio 3.0, you can set up a fast PCR or conventional PCR (standard PCR) as per software available in instrument (Table 4).

Funding

This work was partially funded by American Heart Association's Transformational Project Award 23TPA1140823, Innovative Project Grant 23IPA105444, and National Institutes of Health R01 grant HL164794 and startup funds from the Temple University to V.N.S.G. AKR is supported with the American Heart Association-Post Doctoral Fellowship grant 2021AHA000POST000217114.

References

1. Garikipati VNS et al (2019) Circular RNA CircFndc3b modulates cardiac repair after myocardial infarction via FUS/VEGF-A axis. Nat Commun 10(1):4317
2. Rai AK et al (2021) Decoding the complexity of circular RNAs in cardiovascular disease. Pharmacol Res 171:105766
3. Rai AK et al (2021) Current status and potential therapeutic strategies for using non-coding RNA to treat diabetic cardiomyopathy. Front Physiol 11:612722
4. Kristensen LS et al (2019) The biogenesis, biology and characterization of circular RNAs. Nat Rev Genet 20(11):675–691
5. Salzman J et al (2013) Cell-type specific features of circular RNA expression. PLoS Genet 9(9):e1003777

6. Westholm JO et al (2014) Genome-wide analysis of drosophila circular RNAs reveals their structural and sequence properties and age-dependent neural accumulation. Cell Rep 9(5):1966–1980
7. Chen H-H et al (2022) Circular RNA detection identifies circ PSEN1 alterations in brain specific to autosomal dominant Alzheimer's disease. Acta Neuropathol Commun 10(1):29
8. Patil NS et al (2021) Circular RNA mediated gene regulation in chronic diabetic complications. Sci Rep 11(1):23766
9. Vo JN et al (2019) The landscape of circular RNA in cancer. Cell 176(4):869–881. e13
10. Amaya L et al (2023) Circular RNA vaccine induces potent T cell responses. Proc Natl Acad Sci 120(20):e2302191120
11. Chen R et al (2023) Engineering circular RNA for enhanced protein production. Nat Biotechnol 41(2):262–272
12. Kameda S, Ohno H, Saito H (2023) Synthetic circular RNA switches and circuits that control protein expression in mammalian cells. Nucleic Acids Res 51(4):e24–e24
13. Wu W, Zhao F, Zhang J (2023) circAtlas 3.0: a gateway to 3 million curated vertebrate circular RNAs based on a standardized nomenclature scheme. Nucleic Acids Res 52:gkad770
14. Das A, Das D, Panda AC (2022) Validation of circular RNAs by PCR. Methods Mol Biol 2392:103–114
15. Pandey PR et al (2019) RPAD (RNase R treatment, polyadenylation, and poly (A)+ RNA depletion) method to isolate highly pure circular RNA. Methods 155:41–48
16. Vromman M et al (2022) CIRCprimerXL: convenient and high-throughput PCR primer design for circular RNA quantification. Front Bioinf 2:834655

Chapter 12

Identification and Analysis of Small Nucleolar RNAs by Real-Time Quantitative PCR

Amit Kumar Rai, Tiffany Lee, and Venkata Naga Srikanth Garikipati

Abstract

One of the greatest scientific achievements of the twenty-first century is the completion of The Human Genome Project (HGP). Thereafter, we came to know that the human genome codes nearly 2% for making proteins and thus named as coding genes, suggesting the rest of the genome as noncoding or junk. However, research in the past two decades has shown and established that noncoding RNAs are major contributors of regulating and modulating the various function of cells as well as tissues. Noncoding RNAs can be classified as basis of their sizes in two categories, long noncoding RNAs (>200 nt) and small noncoding RNAs (<200 nt). Small nucleolar RNAs (snoRNAs) are part of the small noncoding RNA family and primarily reside inside the nucleus of eukaryotes. Sno RNAs can be divided into two major categories based on their distinguished structure and function; these are C/D box and HACA box snoRNAs. They participate in the posttranscriptional modifications on ribosomal RNAs (r-RNAs), transfer RNAs (t-RNAs), messenger RNAs (m-RNAs), and small nuclear RNAs (snRNAs). Sno RNAs act as guide RNAs to modify other noncoding RNAs by pseudouridylation or 2′O ribomethylation. We discussed in this protocol about one of the widely used techniques for detection and analysis of snoRNAs, i.e., real-time quantitative PCR (RT-qPCR).

Key words Small nucleolar RNA, Real-time qPCR, TaqMan or SYBR chemistry detection method, Pseudouridylation, 2′O methylation

1 Introduction

The Human Genome Project, which began in 1990 and concluded in 2003, pioneered the analysis and sequencing of the 92% of human genome [1–3]. Recently, with the advancement of technology, we got to know the full sequence of human genome [4]. Afterward, it was discovered that nearly 2% of the genome encodes for proteins, and the remaining 98% was considered as noncoding. In the past two decades, researchers reported these noncoding RNAs play a major role in regulation of function of cells in various diseases, including cardiovascular diseases (CVDs) [5–7].

Dhananjie N. K. Chandrasekera and Rajesh Katare (eds.), *Cardiomyocytes: Methods and Protocols*, Methods in Molecular Biology, vol. 2894, https://doi.org/10.1007/978-1-0716-4342-6_12,

In this chapter, we will focus on a specific type of noncoding RNA. Small nucleolar RNAs (snoRNAs) are a class of noncoding RNAs found in the nucleolus of cells that direct chemical modifications of other RNAs, such as ribosomal RNAs (rRNAs) and small nuclear RNAs (snRNAs) [8]. SnoRNA can be classified into two classes: C/D box (SNORD) or H/ACA box (SNORA), which are characterized by conserved sequences of nucleic acids, or boxes [5]. snoRNAs are known to guide 2′-O-methylation, which is the addition of a methyl group to the 2′ hydroxyl of the ribose sugar in the RNA backbone, and pseudouridylation, the conversion of uridine to pseudouridine. Eukaryotic snoRNAs are commonly found within the introns of both coding and noncoding genes. Additionally, some snoRNAs are transcribed by RNA polymerase II from specific snoRNA loci in the genome [5]. In recent years, snoRNA has exhibited abilities to serve as potential disease biomarkers [5]. Real-time quantitative PCR (RT-qPCR) is a widely used technique for identification and analysis of snoRNAs.

2 Materials

We summarize the procedure necessary to identify snoRNAs in cells and tissues (such as the heart) as follows (Fig. 1).

2.1 RNA Isolation and Quantification

- miRNeasy tissue/cells advanced mini kit (Cat # 217604, Qiagen, USA) (*see* **Note 1**).
- Ethanol for molecular biology.
- 4 °C microcentrifuge (*see* **Note 2**).

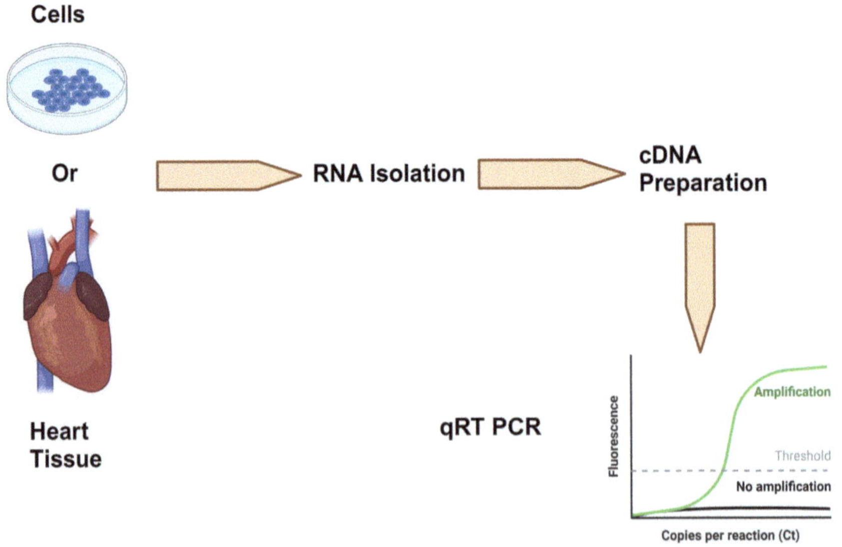

Fig. 1 Schematic representations of steps involved in identification of snoRNAs by real-time quantitative PCR

- Mini vortexer (*see* **Note 2**).
- Accu-jet pro pipette (*see* **Note 2**).
- NanoDrop One spectrophotometer.
- Nuclear-free tips including 10 μL, 20–200 μL, 1000 μL (*see* **Note 2**).
- Ultrapure nuclease-free water (*see* **Note 2**).

2.2 cDNA Preparation and Real-Time PCR

- High-capacity c-DNA reverse transcription kit (Cat #4368814, Applied Biosystems, USA) (*see* **Note 3**).
- Mini Amp Thermal Cycler (*see* **Note 2**).
- QuantStudio real-time PCR system (QuantStudio 3.0, Applied Biosystems, USA) (*see* **Notes 2** and **4**).
- MicroAmp Fast 96-well reaction plate (0.1 mL or 0.2 mL) (*see* **Note 4**).
- MicroAmp optical adhesive film.
- Filter pipette tips.
- Microcentrifuge tube.
- PlateFuge™ Microplate Microcentrifuge with rotor and plate carrier.

3 Methods

In the following protocol, all necessary steps should be performed at room temperature unless stated otherwise.

3.1 Primer Designing

To design the primer specific to any snoRNA, we will follow the convergent method of designing primers.

3.2 RNA Isolation

RNA isolation for identification of snoRNAs can be performed as per requirement of the experiments in the cell cultures or tissues. We outlined the procedures as follows:

1. Follow the manufacturer's protocol for RNA isolation (miR-Neasy tissue/cells advanced mini kit, Cat # 217604, Qiagen, USA). Before starting the RNA isolation, reconstitute all the buffers as directed in the handbook of this kit. Keep all the buffers at room temperature. This method of RNA isolation will provide total RNA as well as small size RNAs (<200 nt).
2. Homogenize 30 mg of frozen tissue or 1×10^7 cells in 260 μL of RLT buffer. For homogenization of cells/tissues, any process can be used such as syringe needle or tissue rupture II (*see* **Note 5**).

3. After homogenization of cells/tissues, add 80 μL of buffer AL (provided with kit) and mix well by pipetting or vortexing. Keep the samples at room temperature for 3 min.
4. After 3 min of incubation with AL buffer, transfer the lysates into a genomic DNA eliminator column (provided with kit) and centrifuge at 8000× *g* for 30 s. Make sure all the liquids come into the collection tube, if not then centrifuge again.
5. If working with animal tissues, add 20 μL of RPP buffer, vortex it, and keep for 3 min at room temperature (*see* **Note 6**). Then, centrifuge for 3 min at 12,000× *g* to precipitate the pellet. Transfer the supernatant into a fresh 2.0 mL tube.
6. Add 1 volume of isopropanol to the 2.0 mL tube and mix by pipetting. Transfer 700 μL of volume from previous steps to a fresh RNeasy mini column and centrifuge for 30 s at 8000× *g*. Discard the flow-through and reuse the column and collection tube if using more than 700 μL of volume.
7. In the following steps, add the buffers (RWT and RPE) as 700 μL and 500 μL as per directed by the manufacturer and centrifuge for 30 s at 8000× *g*. Discard the flow-through and transfer the column to a new collection tube (*see* **Note 7**).
8. Add 80% ethanol (500 μL) to the RNeasy mini column and centrifuge at 8000× *g* for 3 min. Remove the column and keep in another collection tube, and place in centrifuge for 1 min at 15,000× *g* to make sure there is no more ethanol left in the column.
9. Take out the dry column from centrifuge and put it in a 1.5 mL tube (supplied with kit). Add 25–30 μL of RNase-free water (supplied with kit) in the column and centrifuge for 1 min at full speed.
10. This eluted RNA can be quantified immediately on nano drop or can be stored in a deep freezer (−20 °C or − 80 °C) for long-term storage.

3.3 cDNA Synthesis

1. For cDNA synthesis, carry out the following steps as per directed by manufacturer's protocol (high-capacity c-DNA Reverse transcription kit (Cat #4368814, Applied Biosystems, USA). This recommended kit can be used up to 2 μg of RNA to make cDNA in 20 μL of reaction (*see* **Note 8**).
2. Keep all the components of the cDNA synthesis kit on ice to thaw, except enzyme (*see* **Note 9**).
3. Set the reaction volume as per required (we refer a 20 μL of reaction volume) (Table 1).
4. Keep the cDNA synthesis reactions in a thermal cycler (Table 2).

Table 1
The ingredients and essential amounts required for cDNA synthesis in 20 μL reaction mixture

Ingredients	Amount required (for 20 μL reaction mixture)
10× RT buffer	2.0 μL
100 mM dNTP	0.8 μL
10× random primer	2.0 μL
MultiScribe reverse transcriptase enzyme	1.0 μL
RNase inhibitor	1.0 μL
Nuclease-free water	3.2 μL
Total = 20 μL	**10.0 μL + 10 μL of RNA**

Table 2
The incubation of RNA at different temperatures and time for cDNA synthesis

Incubation	Step 1	Step 2	Step 3	Step 4
Temperature (°C)	25	37	85	4
Time (minutes)	10	120	5	Hold

Table 3
Ingredients of SYBR green chemistry for setting up RT-qPCR

Ingredients	Volume (10 μL/well)	Volume (20 μL/well)
Power up SYBR master mix (2×)	5.0 μL	10.0 μL
Forward primer and reverse primer	0.5–1.0 μM	0.5–1.0 μM
Template cDNA	1 ng–10 ng	1 ng–10 ng
Nuclease-free water	Enough to fill to 10.0 μL	Enough to fill to 20.0 μL
Total	**10.0 μL**	**20.0 μL**

3.4 Identification of snoRNAs by RT-qPCR

1. Synthesized cDNA from the previous section will serve as a template for identification of desired snoRNA.
2. Use snoRNA primers to set up the RT-qPCR (*see* **Note 10**).
3. Set up the reaction as listed in Table 3 as per requirement like triplicate or tetraplicate.
4. Seal the plate with an optical adhesive film and spin it in a microplate microcentrifuge.
5. Set the reaction in QuantStudio 3 and load the plate. Select the protocol for SYBR chemistry (*see* **Note 11**).

3.5 Analysis of q-PCR Data

1. Analysis can be performed by utilizing the cycle threshold (Ct) from QuantStudio 3.0, using $2^{e\ (\Delta\text{-Ct})}$ method for quantification.
2. U6 snRNA primer is widely used as a housekeeping control noncoding RNA (*see* **Note 12**).

4 Notes

1. This kit is good for 50 reactions and contains all the required buffers and columns to eliminate genomic DNA contamination. Please refer to the quick protocol and handbook before starting the experiment.
2. Equipment such as centrifuges, vortexes, pipettes, pipettes tips, thermal cyclers, or QuantStudio 3 listed in this protocol are just examples. You may use any similar products or instruments that suit to follow the essential steps.
3. This kit is good for 200 reactions in 20 μL volume and can be used for 2 μg of RNA to make cDNA.
4. Please pay attention to the block size (0.1 mL or 0.2 mL) when using the QuantStudio 3. You may need to use 96-well PCR plates according to the available block size.
5. Volume of RLT buffer can be adjusted as per amount of tissue or cell.
6. For RNA isolation from the cells, this step is not required.
7. Please make sure to dissolve RWT and RPE buffers as per direction of the manufacturer.
8. This contains all the required items for cDNA synthesis including dNTPs, reverse transcriptase enzyme, primers, RNase inhibitor, and buffers.
9. Maxima reverse transcriptase enzyme can be used directly taking out from freezer.
10. Primers can be designed by utilizing any online primer designing tools such as Primer 3 Plus or can be ordered from other sources such as IDT or Thermo Fisher Scientific.
11. You can choose either fast or standard PCR protocol in QuantStudio 3 software.
12. If a given snoRNA can guide modifications on U6, it is appropriate to choose another internal control.

Funding

This work was partially funded by NIH-R01 HL16479, American Heart Association's Innovative project grant 23IPA105444, as well as startup funds from the Temple University to V.N.S.G. AKR was supported with the American Heart Association-Post Doctoral Fellowship grant 915681.

References

1. Olson MV (1993) The human genome project. Proc Natl Acad Sci USA 90(10):4338–4344
2. Lander ES et al (2001) Initial sequencing and analysis of the human genome. Nature 409(6822):860–921
3. Venter JC et al (2001) The sequence of the human genome. Science 291(5507): 1304–1351
4. Nurk S et al (2022) The complete sequence of a human genome. Science 376(6588):44–53
5. Jagielski NP et al (2024) A contemporary review of snoRNAs in cardiovascular health: RNA modification and beyond. Mol Ther Nucleic Acids 35(1):102087
6. Rai AK et al (2022) Spaceflight-associated changes of snoRNAs in peripheral blood mononuclear cells and plasma exosomes-a pilot study. Front Cardiovasc Med 9:886689
7. Rai AK et al (2020) Current status and potential therapeutic strategies for using non-coding RNA to treat diabetic cardiomyopathy. Front Physiol 11:612722
8. Bratkovic T, Bozic J, Rogelj B (2020) Functional diversity of small nucleolar RNAs. Nucleic Acids Res 48(4):1627–1651

Chapter 13

Extraction of Total Protein from Cardiomyocytes and Western Blotting Analysis

James A. Loehr, Heidy K. Latchman, Robyn M. Murphy, and Tanya R. Cully

Abstract

Using total protein lysates for Western blotting confers greater benefits than traditional approaches that use fractionated samples, where a portion of the sample is discarded during processing. By incorporating low-volume inputs, it is possible to identify any protein present in the sample where a suitable antibody is available. The inclusion of a calibration curve allows quantitative analyses to be undertaken. There are additional benefits including that only requiring a small input saves on precious samples. Using whole muscle lysates is necessary in order to ascertain specificity of antibodies for subsequent immunofluorescent methods.

Key words Western blotting, Whole muscle/tissue lysates, Quantitative analysis

1 Introduction

Western blotting is a technique often utilized to provide information on potential functional and mechanistic impacts of different experimental parameters. However, Western blot data are different between research groups, suggesting they are difficult to replicate. They are often reported in publications with sparse details on how they were performed. In the method presented in this chapter, we reinforce key concepts that should be considered when performing Western blotting. In summary, these are (i) correct solution choice for sample preparation, (ii) no loss of sample during sample preparation, (iii) antibody validation, and (iv) the use of calibration curves being required for quantitative analysis. Importantly, for the latter point, small sample amounts are used to ensure linearity in detection across a dynamic detection range suitable for a given study [1].

Dhananjie N. K. Chandrasekera and Rajesh Katare (eds.), *Cardiomyocytes: Methods and Protocols*, Methods in Molecular Biology, vol. 2894, https://doi.org/10.1007/978-1-0716-4342-6_13,

2 Materials

Prepare all solutions using ultrapure water (prepared by purifying deionized water, to attain a sensitivity of 18 MΩ-cm at 25 °C) and analytical grade reagents. Prepare and store all reagents at room temperature (unless indicated otherwise). Follow all waste disposal regulations when disposing of waste materials.

2.1 Tissue Lysis Buffer Preparation

We recommend that the lysis buffer mimics the intracellular environment of a rested striated muscle cell with regard to ionic strength, osmolality, pH, and resting calcium concentration. Our recommended solution contains 36 m M Na^+, 126 m M K^+, 25 mM EGTA, 90 mM HEPES, 1 mM free Mg^{2+} (10.3 mM total Mg), pH 7.10 with a protease/phosphatase inhibitor cocktail (*see* **Note 1**).

2.2 Stain-Free SDS Polyacrylamide Gel

SDS gels of a percent acrylamide suitable for the separation of the protein of interest: Bio-Rad prepared stain-free TGX gels in Mini-protean or Criterion (Midi) format or pour your own stain-free gels (*see* **Note 2**). Mini gels allow up to 15 lanes and Midi gels up to 26 lanes.

SDS-PAGE electrophoresis buffer: 0.025 M Tris–HCl, pH 8.3, 0.192 M glycine, 0.1% SDS (*see* **Note 3**).

Denaturing solution (also known as sample buffer or 3 × SDS loading buffer): containing 0.125 M Tris–Cl, pH 6.8, 4% SDS, 10% glycerol, 4 M urea, 10% beta-mercaptoethanol (can be replaced with 15 mM dithiothreitol, DTT), and 0.001% bromophenol blue.

Tris–HCl pH 6.8 solution (*see* **Note 4**).

Bio-Rad Mini-protean or Criterion electrophoresis tanks.

Stained molecular weight marker.

2.3 Immunoblotting

Nitrocellulose or PVDF membranes can be used, and the standard pore size is 0.25 μm. For proteins less than 15 kDa in size, small pore 0.1 μm should be used (*see* **Note 5**).

Filter paper (thickness 0.84 mm). Manufacturer's instructions should be followed as different cassettes require different amounts of filter paper of the given thickness. The end point is a very firm sandwich prepared in a special transfer cassette (see below):

Western blot transfer buffer: 0.025 M Tris–HCl, 0.192 M glycine, 20% methanol (*see* **Note 6**).

Tris-buffered saline (TBS; 10×): 1.5 M NaCl, 0.1 M Tris–HCl, pH 7.4.

Tris-buffered saline with 0.1% Tween 20 (TBST) (*see* **Note 7**).

Blocking solution: Bio-Rad EveryBlot blocking buffer (*see* **Note 8**).

Bio-Rad Mini-protean or Criterion blotting tanks.

2.4 Antibody Probing

Primary and secondary antibodies, diluted in Bio-Rad EveryBlot (*see* **Note 9**).

ECL reagent for horse radish peroxidase (HRP) tagged secondary antibodies. If using fluorescent secondaries, no developing reagent is required (*see* **Note 10**).

3 Methods

3.1 Sample Preparation

1. Quickly and accurately weigh a small portion of frozen whole muscle (5–30 mg; *see* **Note 11**), and place in cold tissue lysis solution at (1:20 wet tissue weight (mg): volume (μL)) on ice. This will give a concentration of 50 μg wet weight tissue/μL.
2. Homogenize tissue (e.g., polytron homogenizer) in 10 s bursts with 30 s rest periods. Keep tube on ice between bursts to prevent sample overheating. Repeat up to three times. Do not centrifuge or boil sample (*see* **Note 12**).
3. Immediately following homogenization, add 3 × SDS denaturing solution (1:2) which will dilute the homogenate to 33 μg. μL^{-1} muscle wet weight.
4. Further dilute the denatured samples to 2.5 μg wet weight muscle·μL^{-1} using 1 × SDS denaturing solution (3 x SDS diluted 2:1 with 1× Tris·Cl pH 6.8) [2].
5. An aliquot from each sample should be combined to generate a sample mix for use as the calibration curve. The volume made should be adequate to load a four-point calibration curve, spanning 3–60 μg of total muscle wet weight (equating to ~1–15 ug total muscle protein) across all the gels that are anticipated for a given study (*see* **Note 13**).

3.2 SDS-PAGE Electrophoresis

1. Clamp and seal the two gels securely to the electrode assembly and place into electrophoresis tanks. If only one gel is being used, a buffer dam replaces the second gel to contain the buffer between the gels separate from the outer chamber. Add electrophoresis buffer to fill the inner chamber (between the gels), so the wells are covered and to ~1 cm above the base of the outer chamber (outside of the gel/electrode assembly). Carefully remove the combs from the gels, avoiding ripping the lanes. Solution should fill the wells.
2. Load 3–5 μL of a standard protein ladder in the first and last lanes of the stain-free gel, the four-point calibration curve, and the samples.
3. Perform electrophoresis at 200 V for 45 min to 1 h, the time is dependent on the percentage of the gel, and until the dye front is just exiting the gel.

4. Following electrophoresis, open the gel plates, carefully remove the gel, and place in a container with cold 1× transfer buffer.
5. Detect the total protein in the gel using UV activation in a Chemidoc imager (Bio-Rad) and by following the manufacturer's protocol (*see* **Note 14**). Select "activate the stain-free gel" (45 s for precast, 5 min for handcast) and auto expose the gel. Ensure highlight saturated pixels has been selected to avoid saturation of any protein bands within the sample lanes. If required, change auto exposure time to obtain a non-saturated image .
6. Cut nitrocellulose or PVDF membranes to fit the gel size. If using PVDF, activate it in methanol for 10 min before equilibrating in cold 1× transfer buffer. Notch top right corner for orientation of the membrane. Label the membrane with pencil in the top left-hand corner, in an area that is clear of protein being transferred.

3.3 Blot Transfer (See Note 15)

1. Pre-soak blot sponges and filter paper (*see* **Note 16**) in cold 1× transfer buffer.
2. Assemble the Western blot transfer cassette (Fig. 1). With the red side of the cassette down, place a sponge, the appropriate number of pre-wet filter paper (two filter papers on each side for mini protean, one filter paper on each side for Criterion), and using clean gloves and clean plastic forceps, carefully lay the nitrocellulose or PVDF membrane on top of the filter paper. Orientate the notch in the membrane to the top right-hand side of the gel (*see* **Note 16**).
3. Carefully place the SDS-PAGE gel on top of the membrane.

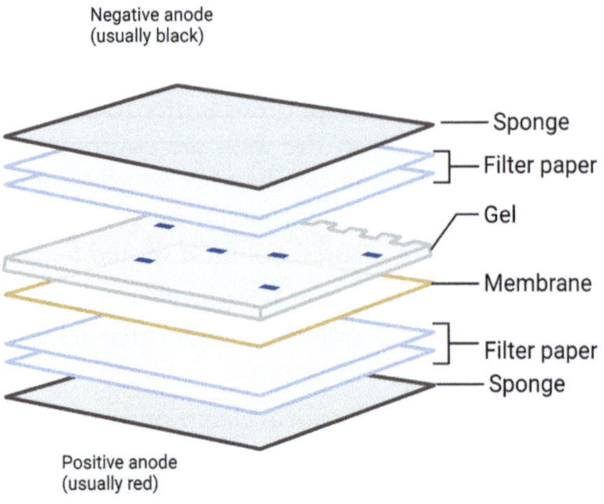

Fig. 1 Western blot transfer cassette assembly

4. Ensure there are no air bubbles between the membrane and gel by gentle rolling, using a gel roller or a smooth glass pipette.
5. Complete the sandwich assembly by adding a filter paper and sponge.
6. Close the gel cassette tightly and insert into the transfer tank with the correct orientation to the electrode. Fill the tank with cold 1× transfer buffer. Add a magnetic stirrer bar to the tank and insert an icepack in the appropriate position at the rear of the sandwich cassettes (*see* **Note 17**).
7. Place the filled tank, with lid, on top of a magnetic stirrer and perform electrophoretic transfer with gentle stirring for either 100 V for 1 h at room temperature for the mini transblot or 100 V for 30 min at room temperature for the Criterion transblot (*see* **Note 18**).
8. Post-transfer, disassemble the transfer cassette, using forceps, place the membrane in TBS, and gently place the gel in a container with used transfer buffer or TBS.
9. Image both the post-transfer gel and membrane on the Chemidoc under stain-free settings, and additional UV activation is not required.

3.4 Antibody Probing

1. If using nitrocellulose membrane, incubating in Miser (Thermo Fisher Scientific), an antibody extending solution, can assist with using less primary antibody.
2. Block the membrane in Bio-Rad EveryBlot on a rocker with gentle rocking for 5 min (*see* **Note 19**).
3. Wash the membrane in TBST for 2 min, and then discard the solution.
4. Incubate the membrane in a primary antibody (diluted in EveryBlot), for 1–2 h at room temperature (*see* **Note 20**) and overnight at 4 °C, all with gentle rocking (*see* **Note 21**).
5. The next day, bring the membrane in the antibody to room temperature on the rocker. Recollect the primary antibody and wash the membrane in TBST for 2 min, 10 min, and 10 min, discarding the solution at each wash step (*see* **Note 22**).
6. Incubate the membrane on the rocker for 1 h in a secondary antibody at room temperature; the secondary antibody concentration used will be dependent on the tag, i.e., HRP fluorescent. Experimental trial starting with manufacturers' recommendations is suggested (*see* **Note 23**).
7. Discard the secondary antibody and wash in TBST for 2 min, 10 min, and 10 min, discarding the solution between each wash (*see* **Note 24**).

8. Use a clean pair of plastic tweezers to take the membrane out of the container and allow excess buffer for drip off. Place the semi-damp membrane on a clean backing, avoiding air bubbles forming underneath.
9. If HRP secondary antibodies are used, apply ECL to the membrane according to the manufacturer's directions and capture images of the standard protein ladder and the detected protein on the membrane (*see* **Note 25**). For fluorescent detection, after washing, place the membrane within the imager and select the appropriate excitation/emission wavelength to capture images for the given secondary antibodies.

3.5 Image Detection

1. Refer to the manufacturer's specifications for the generation or type of imaging machine you are utilizing.
2. Ensure images are acquired at the highest resolution possible.
3. It is best to capture multiple images from faint through to saturated bands.

3.6 Image Analysis

1. Image analysis is performed using Bio-Rad Image Lab software (*see* **Note 26**).
2. To perform quantitative analysis, the stain-free gel and the membrane detected for the protein of interest need to be analyzed. Each will use the calibration curve to determine the relationship between input and output (density).
3. For the stain-free gel, the entire lane density is used. Under the "lanes" tab, manually assign the lane number and adjust and resize the frame as necessary in order to have the entirety of the protein banding within the frame boundaries.
4. Select "lane profile" and check that the rolling ball background subtraction is sufficient.
5. Export the Lane statistics to Excel and use the Adj. Total lane volume (Int) for analysis.
6. Plot the total lane values for the four-point calibration curve as a linear regression and calculate the y-intercept and slope ($y = \text{mx} + c$). Use the equation to solve for the sample (unknown) lanes.
7. Repeat the above steps to analyze proteins of interest detected in the blot image. Ensure you have selected the bands of interest for the given protein.
8. When examining the "lane profile" to ensure the rolling ball background subtraction is sufficient, also check that the peak histogram of the band selection is captured.
9. Select "Analysis table."

10. Under the "Lane and Band" tab, export the band volume intensity measurements to Excel.
11. Plot the volume intensity values for the four-point calibration curve as a linear regression, calculating the y-intercept and slope.
12. To calculate the relative amount of the probed protein to total protein from the calibration curve, use the equation to solve for the unknown ($y = mx + c$), dividing the values from **step 20** by the values in **step 12**.
13. These values can now be graphed in your preferred graphing program (*see* **Note 27**).

4 Notes

1. Utilizing a physiological buffer for lysis, with intracellular levels of Na^+ and K^+, avoids autolysis of proteins and incorrect localization of proteins [3]. In striated muscle, 25 mM EGTA is used to prevent calcium-directed proteolysis [4]. Following homogenization, a solubilizing agent can be added; however, the addition of the 3× SDS denaturing solution provides this as 1% SDS.

   A standard RIPA buffer is not suitable to use because it does not contain K^+ [3].
2. Stain-free technology is used to ensure equal loading and the efficiency of protein transfer. Stain-free technology is advantageous in that it is more sensitive than conventional protein stains, saves time, and allows for total protein normalization, removing the need for a housekeeping protein [5, 6]. There are different forms of stain-free gels; a TGX is the most commonly used. Throughout this protocol, we refer to using Bio-Rad equipment, consumables, and software; any equivalent substitute that has the same capabilities could be utilized but would need to be validated by the user.
3. It is easier to prepare a 10× stock solution of the SDS-PAGE electrophoresis buffer at 250 mM Tris base, 1.92 M glycine, 1% SDS, pH 8.3 ((Tris base: 30.30 g, Glycine: 144.10 g, SDS: 10.00 g, diH2O to 1 L. Do not adjust the pH (~pH 8.3 depending on the Tris and glycine used)). Prepare the 1× stock by measuring 900 mL of diH20 and then adding 100 mL of the 10× SDS-PAGE running buffer stock diH20. Add in this order to minimize foaming of the SDS.
4. 4× $TrisCl^-$ (1.5 M) pH 6.8100 mL: Tris base 0.5 M 6.05 g. Make 80 mL with diH2O. Adjust to pH 6.8 with 10 M HCl. Make 100 mL by adding diH2O. Keep at room temperature.

5. PVDF is a less costly membrane and is useful when multiple probes are required as it is more durable. Downsides are that it requires 10 min of methanol activation, and it has an increased background. For fluorescent secondary antibodies, a low fluorescence PVDF is required should PVDF be preferred. Nitrocellulose is advantageous because of uniform low background, including when using fluorescent secondary antibodies.
6. Prepare a 10× stock solution of transfer buffer, without methanol at 250 mM Tris, 1.92 M glycine (Tris base, 30.30 g; glycine, 144.10 g; diH2O to 1 L). Prepare the 1× transfer buffer by first adding 700 mL diH20, 100 mL of 10× transfer buffer, and 200 mL of methanol. The pH will range from 8.1 to 8.5 depending on the Tris, glycine, and methanol used. This range is suitable and the pH of the solution does not need to be measured/adjusted.
7. In 900 mL of diH20, add 100 mL of the 10× Tris-buffered saline and 1 mL of Tween-20 detergent.
8. A number of different blocking agents are available and suitable to use. Commonly, these are 4% bovine serum albumin (BSA) or skim milk powder prepared at 5% weight to volume in TBST. Batch-to-batch variability with the skim milk powder may introduce variation.
9. Bio-Rad EveryBlot blocking buffer in our hands has been found to be suitable for 99% of proteins analyzed. A good starting dilution is often 1 in 1000 for primary antibodies, but dilution ranges can vary widely, and suppliers' information should be followed in the first instance. Secondary antibodies vary depending on the secondary tag (e.g. HRP, fluorophore, colorimetric), the efficacy of the primary antibody, and the sensitivity of the detection reagent. We recommend using a lower secondary concentration and increasing if the signal is too faint. If too much secondary antibody is used, then "negative" bands can appear (giving the appearance of white or light gray bands on a dark background), or bands can be burned into the membrane and so the procedure must be started from the beginning.
10. Fluorescent secondaries provide the ability to detect multiple targets without interference of previous probes. They are also more sensitive in protein detection with a greater linear dynamic range [7].
11. The size of the tissue will be determined by the amount of sample available and the minimum volume capacity of the homogenization probe being utilized.
12. Keeping the sample unfractionated, i.e., not centrifuging it, avoids problems with quantifying the abundance of your protein of interest (POI) as well as allowing for the visualization of

the specificity of antibodies used in Immunofluorescence (where all sample proteins are present).

13. Prepare sufficient sample homogenate mix for use for all calibration curves across all gels performed for the entire study allowing comparisons of all samples across different gels.
14. UV activation of the stain-free gel ensures transfer of the stain-free moiety to the membrane during blotting. This means the stain-free bands can be visualized to ensure transfer of protein to the membrane. The total protein image is used to quantify the total protein in the sample.
15. For efficient and robust transfer of all molecular weight proteins, wet transfer of proteins is recommended.
16. Filter paper thickness is 0.84 mm. Follow the manufacturer's specification for the generation blotting system you use. In general, Bio-Rad mini protean blotting systems require two filter papers on either side of the transfer sandwich (*see* Fig. 1) and the larger Midi or Criterion blotting systems require one filter paper on each side.
17. It is essential that the gel and the membrane are placed on the correct side of the transfer sandwich so that the electrophoretic transfer occurs in the desired direction, from the gel onto the membrane.
18. Transfer tanks can accommodate two sandwich cassettes, with an ice block inserted at the rear of the unit. Keeping the transfer setup cool is important for successful and even distribution of protein transfer.
19. When performing electrophoretic transfer at 100 V, if the transblot system possesses wire electrodes, then the transfer will require 1 h. If the transblot system has electrode plates, then 30 min is sufficient.
20. The 1–2 h room temperature incubation can be before or after the overnight incubation.
21. Blocking removes nonspecific sites on the membrane, which is those remaining sites that did not have protein transferred to it. If a different blocking reagent is to be used, such as those mentioned in **Note 8**, then the appropriate time for application must be determined.
22. The primary antibody can be used up to four to six times, by adding 0.02% sodium azide as a preservative.
23. Gentle rocking is better than agitation for uniform coverage of antibody over the membrane. It is essential that antibodies are validated to ensure they detect the correct band(s) of interest (*see* [2, 8–10]) and the appropriate working concentration of

the antibody is determined (*see* **Note 9**). The duration of application can also be explored.

24. Secondary antibodies cannot be kept as sodium azide interferes with the HRP tag.
25. The secondary antibody will be raised in a species different from the samples being analyzed and targeted to the species the primary antibody was raised in.
26. Bio-Rad Image Lab software for density analysis is free to download and use from the Bio-Rad website. By using Bio-Rad's software, it is possible to utilize and analyze both the stain-free gel and the blot image of protein samples. If you have used an alternative imaging machine or technique to obtain your images, if these images are exported as a .tif image, they can be read into Image Lab and analyzed as described in this protocol.
27. Do not normalize the protein in a Western blot back to a single control lane (as is often advised in technical bulletins), as this has the potential to bias data. Any control should be run in triplicate. In the method presented, the four-point calibration curve is used as the control across multiple gels in a given study.

Acknowledgements

Figure 1 was generated using BioRender software. The authors have no conflicts of interest to disclose.

References

1. Edwards JN, Friedrich O, Cully TR, von Wegner F, Murphy RM, Launikonis BS (2010) Upregulation of store-operated Ca2+ entry in dystrophic mdx mouse muscle. Am J Physiol Cell Physiol 299(1):C42–C50. https://doi.org/10.1152/ajpcell.00524.2009
2. Murphy RM (2011) Enhanced technique to measure proteins in single segments of human skeletal muscle fibers: fiber-type dependence of AMPK-alpha1 and -beta1. J Appl Physiol 110(3):820–825. https://doi.org/10.1152/japplphysiol.01082.2010
3. Wette SG, Lamb GD, Murphy RM (2023) Calpain-3 is not a sodium dependent protease and simply requires calcium for activation. Int J Mol Sci 24(11). https://doi.org/10.3390/ijms24119405
4. Murphy RM, Dutka TL, Horvath D, Bell JR, Delbridge LM, Lamb GD (2013) Ca2+-dependent proteolysis of junctophilin-1 and junctophilin-2 in skeletal and cardiac muscle. J Physiol 591(3):719–729. https://doi.org/10.1113/jphysiol.2012.243279
5. Gilda JE, Gomes AV (2013) Stain-free total protein staining is a superior loading control to beta-actin for Western blots. Anal Biochem 440(2):186–188. https://doi.org/10.1016/j.ab.2013.05.027
6. Cully TR, Rodney GG (2020) Nox4 – RyR1 – Nox2: regulators of micro-domain signaling in skeletal muscle. Redox Biol 36:101557. https://doi.org/10.1016/j.redox.2020.101557
7. Taylor SC, Rosselli-Murai LK, Crobeddu B, Plante I (2022) A critical path to producing high quality, reproducible data from quantitative western blot experiments. Sci Rep 12(1):17599. https://doi.org/10.1038/s41598-022-22294-x
8. Murphy RM, Lamb GD (2013) Important considerations for protein analyses using

antibody based techniques: down-sizing Western blotting up-sizes outcomes. J Physiol 591(23):5823–5831. https://doi.org/10.1113/jphysiol.2013.263251
9. Murphy RM, Larkins NT, Mollica JP, Beard NA, Lamb GD (2009) Calsequestrin content and SERCA determine normal and maximal Ca2+ storage levels in sarcoplasmic reticulum of fast- and slow-twitch fibres of rat. J Physiol 587(Pt 2):443–460. https://doi.org/10.1113/jphysiol.2008.163162
10. Larkins NT, Murphy RM, Lamb GD (2012) Absolute amounts and diffusibility of HSP72, HSP25, and alphaB-crystallin in fast- and slow-twitch skeletal muscle fibers of rat. Am J Physiol Cell Physiol 302(1):C228–C239. https://doi.org/10.1152/ajpcell.00266.2011

Chapter 14

Cationic Liposome Formulation by Microfluidics for miRNA Delivery

Matthew Reily-Bell and Rishi Shah

Abstract

MiRNA therapeutics for treatment of cardiovascular disease face several problems with delivery. Encapsulation of miRNA therapeutics in cationic liposomes has shown potential to address many of these concerns with miRNA therapeutic delivery. Here we outline the formulation and characterization of cationic liposomes, capable of encapsulating and delivering miRNA therapeutics to AC16 cardiomyocyte cell lines, by microfluidics.

Key words Cationic, Liposomes, Microfluidics, miRNA therapeutics, Qubit, RNA protection assay, RT-qPCR

1 Introduction

Liposomes are small spherical artificial vesicles that can be formed from a combination of cholesterol and natural nontoxic phospholipids. Liposomes can vary in size from 25 nm to 2.5 μm and have one or more membrane bilayers composed of phospholipids that encapsulate an aqueous core [1, 3]. The potential of liposomes for drug delivery has been recognized since their discovery 1965 by Alec Bangham [5]. Liposome encapsulation technology effectively takes advantage of the impulsive nature in which phospholipids form closed structures when hydrated in an aqueous solution. As such a liposomes' final organization is influenced by types, size, morphology, concentration, and charge of the lipids that make it up. This also means that the properties of the solution they are in also play a role, particularly ionic strength, pH, and temperature. There is also an energy cost to the formation of the spherical shape of liposomes, and so the method by which they are prepared influences how they will form [3]. Many approaches have been

Authors Matthew Reily-Bell and Rishi Shah have equally contributed to this chapter.

Dhananjie N. K. Chandrasekera and Rajesh Katare (eds.), *Cardiomyocytes: Methods and Protocols*, Methods in Molecular Biology, vol. 2894, https://doi.org/10.1007/978-1-0716-4342-6_14,

used historically to create nanoparticles. Here we demonstrate the most recent advancement in these technologies, microfluidics. In the microfluidic method, lipids are dissolved in an alcohol solvent (e.g., methanol) which is then focused between two aqueous buffer streams (e.g., water or citrate buffer) in a microfluidic channel. This generates a hydrodynamic laminar flow and a diffusive mixing at interfaces of the two liquids that favors self-assembly of the lipids into vesicles. This method allows for precise control of the mixing ratios and the flow rates of the liquids enabling the generation of small lipid particles while using solvents with low toxicity. Additionally, post-production treatment such as sonication is not required [3]. An ideal liposome will efficiently encapsulate miRNA therapeutics, have an ideal size for cellular uptake of the liposomes (80–150 nm), be uniform in size, and protect miRNA therapeutics from degradation. Thus, cationic liposomes address many of the difficulties with miRNA therapeutic delivery, namely, degradation of miRNA and efficiency of uptake [2, 4].

2 Materials

Prepare all solutions with DNase- and RNase-free water and analytical grade reagents.

2.1 Cationic Liposome Formulation

A. Distearoylphosphatidylcholine (DSPC), store at −20 °C and seal with parafilm to prevent moisture from getting in.

B. Cholesterol, store at −20 °C and seal with parafilm to prevent moisture from getting in.

C. 1,2-Dioleoyl-3-trimethylammonium propane (DOTAP), store at −20 °C and seal with parafilm to prevent moisture from getting in.

D. 1,2-Distearoyl-sn-glycero-3-phosphoethanolamine-poly(ethylene glycol) (DSPE-PEG), store at −20 °C and seal with parafilm to prevent moisture from getting in.

E. Methanol.

F. 100 mM citrate buffer: 0.0825 M sodium citrate dihydrate, 0.0175 M citric acid.

  (a) Dissolve 0.0825 M of sodium citrate dihydrate and 0.0175 M citric acid in 800 mL of water. Adjust to the desired pH using HCL and then make up to 1 L with water.

G. Syringes, 1 mL and 3 mL.

H. miRNA Mimic (5 nmol).

I. Microfluidic cassette.

J. Sonicating water bath.

K. Precision Nanosystems NanoAssemblr® Benchtop.

2.2 Liposome Characterization

A. 10 kd ultra-centrifugal filters.

B. Eppendorf tubes.

C. Cuvettes for DLS and measuring zeta potential.

D. Zeta sizer or equivalent device.

E. Nano-assembler.

2.3 Measuring miRNA Encapsulation

A. Triton X-100.

B. Qubit miRNA assay kit (*see* **Note 1**).

2.4 RNA Protection Assay

A. TBE buffer: 124 mM Tris base, 125 mM boric acid, and 5 mM EDTA.

   (a) Make a 2.5× TBE buffer stock solution by dissolving 124 mM Tris base, 125 mM boric acid, and 5 mM ethylenediaminetetraacetic acid (EDTA) in distilled water.

   (b) Dilute stock solution 1 in 5 with distilled water to make a 0.5× TBE working solution.

B. Agarose powder,

C. RNase A,

D. Bleach containing 5% sodium hypochlorite by weight and 0.01–0.05% sodium hydroxide (household bleach).

E. SYBR Gold nucleic acid stain.

F. Gel electrophoresis setup.

G. RNase inhibitor.

H. Triton X-100.

I. UV light gel imaging system.

3 Methods

The following is a protocol for the formulation of DOTAP-based cationic liposomes by microfluidics. Carry out all experiments at room temperature unless otherwise specified. Prepare fresh pH 3.5100 mM citrate buffer before each encapsulation. All H_2O is DNase-, RNase-, DNA-, and RNA-free unless otherwise specified. Following use of these protocols, liposomes can be used to treat cell lines using standard transfection protocols following standard cell toxicity assays (*see* **Note 2**).

3.1 Cationic Liposome Formulation

3.1.1 Formulation of Empty Control Liposomes

1. Weigh out 1.96 mg DSPC, 4.64 mg Chol, 6.031 mg DOTAP, and 1 mg DSPE-PEG2000 on nonstick weighing paper. This is a molar ratio of 8.6:40:26:1 for DSPC:CHOL:DOTAP:DSPE-PEG2000. Add these to a tube of at least 2 mL total volume along with 1.4 mL of methanol (*see* **Notes 3–4**). You will now have an 8 mg/mL solution of lipids in methanol; however, these will need to be dissolved (Table 1).

Table 1
Chemicals used in lipid nanoparticle formulation

Chemical	Weight	Molar ratio
DSPC	1.96 mg	8.6
CHOL	4.64 mg	40
DOTAP	6.031 mg	26
DSPE-PEG2000	1 mg	1

2. To dissolve lipids in methanol completely, heat a sonicating water bath to 65 °C and sonicate in 1 min intervals while moving the tube around. Between intervals, invert the tube five to ten times, in order to ensure no lipids are stuck higher up in the tube. After 3 min of sonication, check that no particles are visible in the solution by holding the tube up to a light. Continue to sonicate if not all lipids are dissolved.
3. Equilibrate your microfluidic cassette with your organic solvent. Then set the microfluidic machine to the following parameters: an aqueous to lipid ratio of 5:1, a flow rate of 5 mL/min, and a total volume to be made of 2 mL. Ensure you set the syringe sizes to the size you use to take up your aqueous and lipid phases (*see* **Notes 5–7).**
4. Use a 1 mL syringe to take up your lipids dissolved in methanol and a 3 mL syringe to take up your aqueous buffer (pH 3.5 100 mM citrate buffer). Proceed to formulate your liposomes and collect these in an appropriately sized tube. This formulates empty control liposomes (*see* **Notes 4** and **8**).
5. Before continuing with formulation, measure particle size, PDI, and zeta potential using a zeta sizer (Subheading 3.2, **step 1**). If particle size, PDI, and zeta potential are within the desired parameters, proceed to encapsulate your miRNA (*see* **Note 9**).

3.1.2 Formulation of miRNA-Loaded Liposomes

1. To prepare your miRNA therapeutic for encapsulation, dissolve 5 nmols of miRNA mimics in 50 μL of DNA-, RNA-, DNase-, and RNase-free H_2O. H_2O can be heated to 37 °C to help dissolve the RNA in addition to vortexing the mixture. Store miRNA on ice when not in use. Mix the miRNA mimics in the desired proportions so the that you have a total of 5 nmols in 50 μL.
2. Add 850 μL of pH 3.5 100 mM citrate buffer to the dissolved miRNA mimic bringing the total volume to 900 μL. Take up the miRNA mimic solution in a 1 mL syringe and replace the

previous aqueous phase syringe with it. Run the microfluidic machine and collect the liposomes. Total volume to be made should be 1 mL.

3. Remove the remaining ~100 μL of aqueous buffer from the syringe and store at −20 °C for use in RNA protection assays.
4. Cassettes can be used ~7 times before significant reduction in liposome quality is observed (*see* **Note 10**).

3.2 Liposome Characterization

1. Measure particle size, PDI, and zeta potential in a Malvern zeta sizer or other device capable of measuring dynamic light scattering (DLS). To reduce sample waste, dilute 25 μL of encapsulated liposomes in 1 mL of HPLC water. Reuse the same sample for measuring both size and charge.
2. Liposomes need to be purified before further characterization and use. This can be done either via traditional dialysis or via ultracentrifugation.
   (a) Traditional dialysis should be done at 4 °C overnight against water or PBS. Purification via 10 kD ultracentrifugal filters can be done by equilibrating columns by the addition of 1 mL of water and spinning at 4000× *g* for 5 min; discard both flow through and remaining liquid in the column. Samples should then be diluted 1 in 7 in DNase-, RNase-, and nucleotide-free H_2O and centrifuged at 4000× *g* for 30 min. Discard flow through and aliquot remaining liquid in the column into Eppendorf tubes. There should be less than 2 mL left.
3. Repeat DLS and zeta potential measurements 0, 1, 3, 5, 7, and 10 days after dialysis. 50 μL diluted in 950 H_2O is recommended for this, and then should be kept at 4 °C and reused for each time point (Fig. 1) (*see* **Note 11**).
4. Use cryo-transmission electron microscopy to visualize purified liposomes (Fig. 2) (*see* **Note 12**).

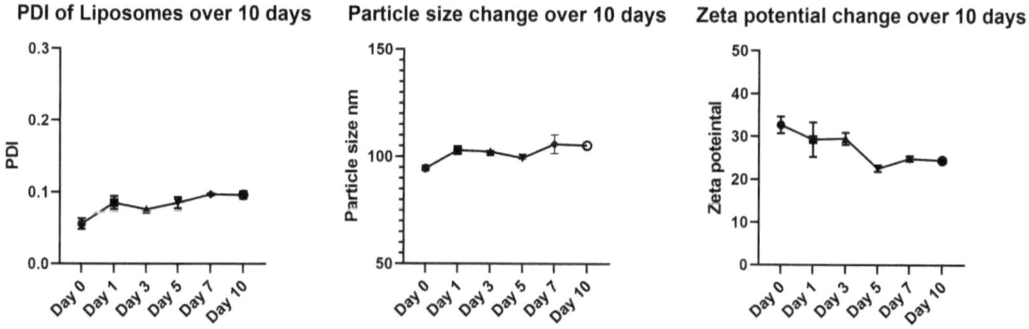

Fig. 1 Particle size, PDI, and zeta potential over 10 days. $N = 3$ separate encapsulation. Lipid nanoparticles were synthesized using the microfluidic protocol outlined in this chapter

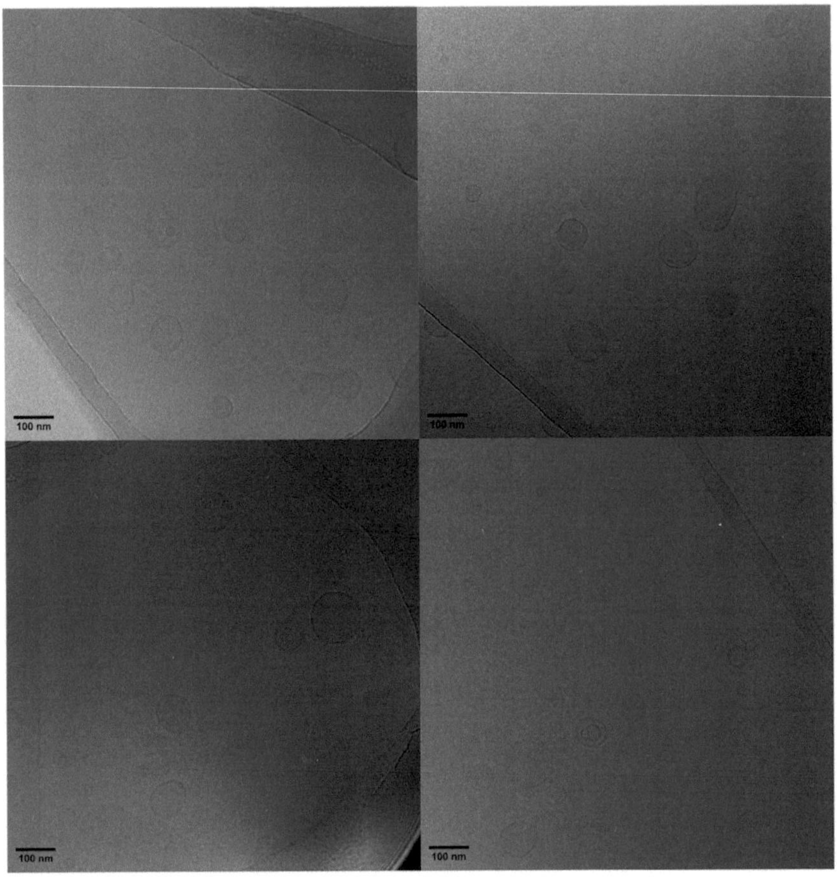

Fig. 2 Cryo-TEM of LNPs. Black rings are lipid membranes surrounding nanoparticles. Images are taken at 50,000× magnification

3.3 Measuring Encapsulation Efficiency via Qubit®

1. Liposomes were lysed by taking 4 μL of liposomes and adding 5 μL 2% Triton X-100 to a PCR tube and making up to 20 μL with DNAse-, RNAse-, and nucleotide-free H_2O.
2. Mix the solution via vortexing or pipetting and then spin down for 3 s.
3. Incubate the solutions at 25°C for 20 min to allow breakdown of the liposomes.
4. Carry out Qubit® miRNA assay according to the manufacturer's instructions except Triton X-100 which should be added to the standards so that the final Triton X-100 concentration is 0.001% (*see* **Note 13**).
5. Results should be multiplied by 5 to account for the dilution of liposomes when lysing using Triton X-100. This is then subsequently multiplied by the number of microliters (μL) obtained after purification to find the total weight of miRNA encapsulated.

6. To convert this weight into nmols, New England Biosciences' Bio Calculator (NEBioCalculator) can be used. Go to RNA Mass to Moles converter and enter the size of our miRNA therapeutic into the RNA length column. Then input the RNA mass calculated from the Qubit measurement (*see* **Note 14**).
7. To calculate encapsulation efficiency, divide the measured encapsulated miRNA by the theoretical maximum encapsulation and multiply by 100% (*see* **Note 15**). To determine the theoretical maximum encapsulation, the following equation can be used:

$$\text{Theoretical Maximum} = \left(\frac{\text{Moles of RNA used}}{\text{The total volume of aqueous phase}}\right) * (\text{The proportion of aqueous phase used}) * \left(\frac{\text{Volume Produced} - (\text{Waste} + \text{The amount of aqueous phase kept asside for DLS and Zeta sizing})}{\text{Volume Produced}}\right)$$

3.4 RNA Protection Assays

In order to assess the ability of the liposomes to protect the miRNA therapeutic, it can be challenged with RNAse A and visualized on a denaturing 1% TBE agarose gel. For this, the following protocol can be used.

3.4.1 Preparation of Denaturing 1% TBE Agarose Gel

1. Weigh 0.5 g of agarose powder and place in a microwave safe container.
2. Add 1 mL of standard bleach and incubate for 2 min.
3. Make the volume up to 50 mL with TBE buffer and microwave in 20 s intervals until all of the agarose powder has been dissolved.
4. Allow the agarose to cool briefly until the container can be picked up.
5. Add 5 μL of SYBR gold nucleic acid stain or equivalent stain and swirl gently (*see* **Note 16**).
6. Pour the molten agarose solution into an appropriate cassette, insert the lane comb, and wait ~30 min for the agarose to set completely.

3.4.2 RNAse Challenge and Liposome Lysis

1. While the agarose gel sets, 200 ng of encapsulated miRNA and 200 ng of unencapsulated miRNA (leftover miRNA in aqueous buffer is good for this) should be aliquoted into two tubes each.
2. To one tube of each encapsulated miRNA and unencapsulated miRNA, add 20 ng RNAse A, and to the others, add an equal volume of RNAse-free H_2O. Mix by vortexing and incubate at 37°C for 30 min.

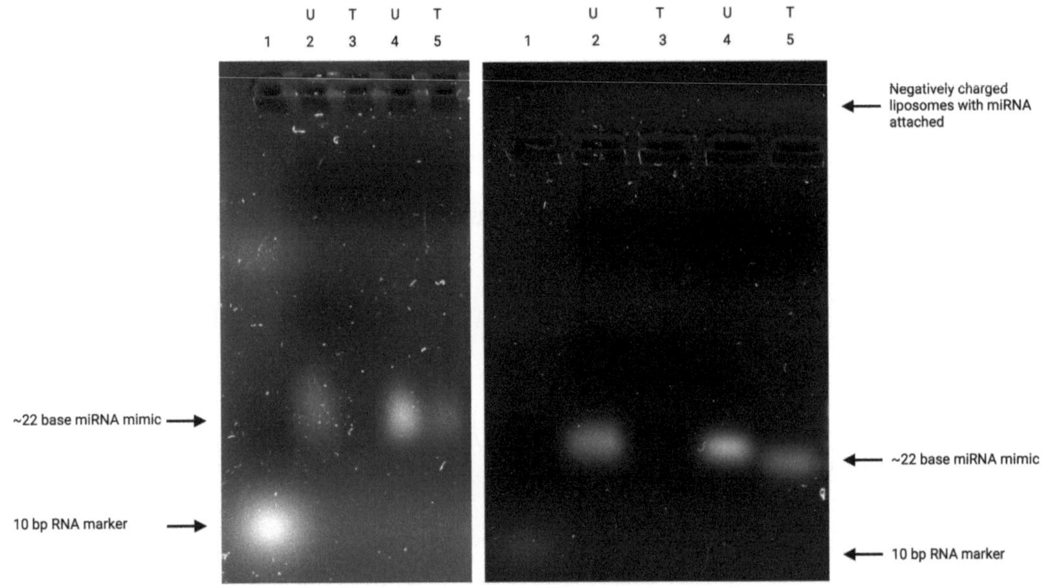

Fig. 3 RNA challenge assay electrophoresis on a 1% HCL 1.5% agarose denaturing gel: (1). RNA marker ladder. (2). Untreated, free-floating miRNA mimic. (3). Free-floating miRNA mimic treated with ten units of RNAse A for 30 min. (4). miRNA mimic from untreated solid lipid nanoparticle. (5). miRNA mimic from a solid lipid nanoparticle, treated with ten units of RNAse A for 30 min

3. Next inactivate RNAse A by adding 20 units of RNAse inhibitor and incubate for 10 min at 25°C.
4. Then add Triton X-100 to samples so that the final concentration of samples is 0.5% Triton X-100. Incubate samples in Triton X-100 for 20 min at 25°C to thoroughly lyse the liposomes.
5. Load samples into the 1% denaturing agarose gel along with a low molecular weight RNA marker ladder and electrophorese at 90 V for ~30 min. Image gels using a UV light imager (Fig. 3).

3.5 Treating AC16 Cells with Cationic Liposomes Containing miRNA Therapeutics

Treatment of AC16 cells can be carried out by simply mixing the liposome treatment with media so that the desired therapeutic concentration is achieved. Normal cell culture media can then be replaced with the new media containing the liposome treatment. Rt-qPCR or droplet digital PCR can be used to measure changes in miRNA levels (Fig. 4).

4 Notes

1. The Qubit® microRNA assay kit is used as this kit tolerates a moderate amount of Triton X-100 in solution which is used to

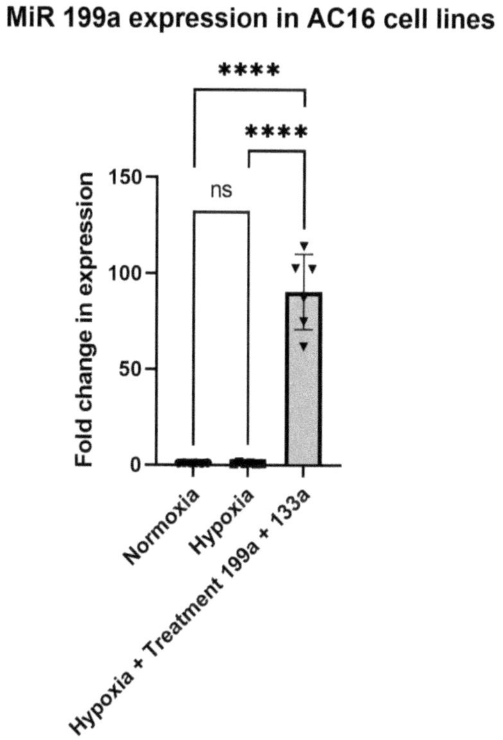

Fig. 4 Changes in miRNA 199a expression after treatment with miRNA 199a mimic-encapsulated in LNPs. Treatment dose was 10 fmol/uL, $N = 6$ biological replicates

lyse the liposomes for miRNA quantification. Other quantification kits such as the commonly used Quant-it™ RiboGreen RNA assay kit can be used; however, we find the qubit miRNA assay kit that uses the same dyes more convenient.

2. Most of the protocol is applicable to other cationic lipid formulations using other lipids such as dimethyldioctadecylammonium (DDA).
3. DOTAP is sticky and will still stick to both the weighing paper and utensils used to move it while weighing. To overcome this, slowly dispense 1.4 mL of methanol onto the filter paper and the utensils while scraping the DOTAP into the tube.
4. PEGylation is essential for reducing particle size with low pH aqueous buffers.
5. Higher flow rates produce smaller particles.
6. Higher A:L ratios have differential effects on particle size and PDI in response to other particle parameters and conditions. A range should be tested for your specific formulation.
7. Higher lipid concentrations reduce particle size.
8. Lower pH citrate buffer reduces particle size.

9. Cationic liposomes formed should be less than 120 nm in size with a PDI less than 0.2 and a zeta potential greater than 10.
10. If planning on encapsulating more than one miRNA mimic cocktail, repeat **step 3** between each new cocktail formulation and discard to remove residual miRNA mimics present in the cassette.
11. DLS and zeta sizing is repeated to ensure that the particle size and charge are stable over time.
12. DOTAP is prone to forming films, so samples should be diluted approximately 1:4 in dH_2O to help with visualization.
13. Triton X-100 can cause skewed reading in a Qubit assay; adding Triton X-100 to the standard improves accuracy of the final readings.
14. The NEBioCalculator will use the average molecular weight of ribonucleotides to estimate the molecular mass of your therapeutic based on its length and then calculate how many moles of your therapeutic are present by dividing the mass of the therapeutic detected by Qubit by the molecular mass of your RNA therapeutic: Mols of miRNA theriputic $= \frac{\mu\text{g RNA measured}}{\frac{\mu\text{g}}{\text{Mol}}\text{ of RNA theriputic}}$
15. Calculation example: $\left(\frac{5\text{ nmol}}{900\ \mu\text{L}}\right) * 833\ \mu\text{L} * \left(\frac{1000\ \mu\text{L} - 275\ \mu\text{L}}{1000\ \mu\text{L}}\right) =$ 3.587 nmol of miRNA therapeutic as the theoretical maximal yield. If the amount encapsulated was 2.344 nmol, then $\left(\frac{2.344\text{ nmol}}{3.587\text{ nmol}}\right) * 100\% = 65.3\%$ encapsulation.
16. Allowing the molten agarose to cool slightly prevents SYBR gold nucleic acid stain vaporizing when it is added. It is however important to add the stain before the molten agarose cools too much; otherwise, clumps of agarose can form and bubbles can be trapped in the agarose when swirling.

References

1. Akbarzadeh A, Rezaei-Sadabady R, Davaran S, Joo SW, Zarghami N, Hanifehpour Y, Samiei M, Kouhi M, Nejati-Koshki K (2013) Liposome: classification, preparation, and applications. Nanoscale Res Lett 8:102
2. Chen S, Tam YYC, Lin PJC, Sung MMH, Tam YK, Cullis PR (2016) Influence of particle size on the in vivo potency of lipid nanoparticle formulations of siRNA. J Control Release 235: 236–244
3. Lombardo D, Kiselev MA (2022) Methods of liposomes preparation: formation and control factors of versatile nanocarriers for biomedical and nanomedicine application. Pharmaceutics 14:543
4. Lou G, Anderluzzi G, Schmidt ST, Woods S, Gallorini S, Brazzoli M, Giusti F, Ferlenghi I, Johnson RN, Roberts CW, O'hagan DT, Baudner BC, Perrie Y (2020) Delivery of self-amplifying mRNA vaccines by cationic lipid nanoparticles: the impact of cationic lipid selection. J Control Release 325:370–379
5. Sessa G, Weissmann G (1968) Phospholipid spherules (liposomes) as a model for biological membranes. J Lipid Res 9:310–318

Chapter 15

Quantification of Sympathetic Nerve Traffic to the Heart: Electrophysiological Recording of Cardiac Sympathetic Nerve Activity in a Rodent Model

Daryl O. Schwenke

Abstract

The accurate measurement of sympathetic nerve activity is essential for advancing knowledge related to the mechanisms that underpin sympathetic activation in diseased states, such as acute heart failure. Considering sympathetic outflow throughout the body is differentially modulated, the most reliable method of measuring sympathetic traffic to individual organs is by way of direct electrophysiological recording of nerve activity. However, the surgical approach of accessing, exposing, and isolating the sympathetic nerve of interest is technically demanding, especially in the small size of a standard laboratory rat, one of the most common models for measuring SNA. Moreover, preserving the health of the nerve while attaching it to electrodes for recording requires careful diligence. The complexity of recording from specifically the cardiac sympathetic nerve remains a significant challenge due to the difficulty of accessing the nerve within the thorax cavity. Here, we describe in detail the process of surgically isolating the cardiac sympathetic nerve activity in a rat for accurately recording and quantifying sympathetic nerve activity.

Key words Cardiac, Sympathetic nerve, Electrophysiology, In vivo model

1 Introduction

The pathological activation of the sympathetic nervous system (SNS) remains one of the most detrimental hallmarks associated with a plethora of cardiovascular morbidities, including heart failure (e.g., myocardial infarction) and systemic hypertension. Determining the efficacy of novel and emerging experimental treatments for ameliorating sympathetic hyperactivation requires a precise measure of sympathetic tone in the first place. Indeed, failure to accurately and selectively measure sympathetic traffic to individual organs of interest, such as the heart following an acute myocardial infarction, risks failing the detection of improvements in sympathetic tone following novel therapeutic intervention.

Dhananjie N. K. Chandrasekera and Rajesh Katare (eds.), *Cardiomyocytes: Methods and Protocols*, Methods in Molecular Biology, vol. 2894, https://doi.org/10.1007/978-1-0716-4342-6_15,

1.1 Differential Outflow of the Sympathetic Nervous System

Although sympathetic outflow ultimately originates from within the rostral ventral lateral medulla of the brainstem, it is well recognized that the SNS is not controlled as a unitary entity, but rather its segmental organization allows for organ-specific responses to be elicited in synchrony [1]. The coordinated changes in sympathetic outflow to specific organs allows selective control of different functions, such as blood pressure and body temperature [2]. Extensive anatomical and neurophysiological evidence supports this organizational model and clearly emphasizes the capacity of the SNS to exert its extrinsic control of organ systems in a highly differential manner [3, 4].

1.2 Methods of Measuring SNA

In light of the differential manner in which SNA is controlled, the method for measuring SNA needs to be carefully considered, as it can impact on the validity of findings and any inferences drawn from them. Clinical studies often quantify global SNA in humans through measurement of plasma or urinary nor-adrenaline (NA) concentration [5]. However, these are widely regarded as nonspecific and highly unreliable indices of SNA [6, 7], due to their poor sensitivity and inability to accurately quantify regional, or organ-specific, SNA.

Heart rate variability (HRV) has been used as a noninvasive predictor of cardiac sympathetic tone [8, 9]. HRV analysis involves assessing the presence of physiological variation in the beat-to-beat interval of HR. From this, the degree of sympathetic and parasympathetic control of the heart can be estimated [10]. However, a major limitation to this technique is that, while low-frequency (~0.1 Hz) variations in HR are thought to be predominantly influenced by sympathetic input, elevations in SNA, such as during cardiac ischemia [11] or exercise conditions [12], are often not depicted in changes to the low-frequency variability.

The most widely accepted "gold-standard" approach for measuring SNA is the use of electrophysiology to directly measure neural electrical activity from the specific sympathetic nerve that is innervating the organ of interest. The procedure involves isolating the sympathetic nerve of interest, placing the nerve across bipolar electrodes, and amplifying and filtering the signal before quantifying the final signal output. In the scientific field, standard laboratory animals have become the most common model for measuring SNA, in particular the lab rat. And while recording activity from renal, lumbar, splenic, and muscle sympathetic nerves are relatively straightforward, due to the ease of accessing and isolating the nerve, recording from the cardiac sympathetic nerve remains a significant challenge due to the difficulty of accessing the nerve within the thorax cavity, without disrupting the natural physiological milieu of the heart and lungs.

Here, an instructional step-by-step guide for recording cardiac SNA in a rat model is presented for those that aim to introduce cardiac sympathetic recording as a routine procedure for investigating, e.g., sympathetic control of the heart following myocardial infarction.

2 Materials

1. Urethane anesthesia (*see* **Note 1**).
2. Custom-made platinum recording electrodes (*see* **Note 2**).
3. Fluid replacement (*see* **Note 3**).
4. Surgical tools:
   (i) Surgical scissors.
   (ii) Micro-scissors.
   (iii) Hemostats (large and small).
   (iv) Straight and curved fine forceps.
   (v) Straight and curved tissue forceps.
   (vi) Bone cutters.
   (vii) Small vessel cauterizer.
5. Consumables:
   (i) Saline.
   (ii) Paper tissues and cotton wool (for mopping up any excess fluid).
   (iii) Paraffin oil (for immersing the nerve preparation).
   (iv) Silk ligature (2–0 and 4–0).
   (v) Compressed oxygen gas (delivered to the inspirate port of the rodent ventilator).

3 Methods

3.1 Surgical Preparation

Anesthesia—Prior to commencing surgery, rats are deeply anesthetized by an intraperitoneal (i.p.) injection of urethane (dose = 1.5 g/kg) (*see* **Note 6**). Despite its carcinogenic properties, urethane is ideal for electrophysiology due to its pharmacologic ability to induce general anesthesia for extended periods of time with relative preservation of respiratory, sympathetic, and cardiovascular reflexes [13].

Once the rat is fully anesthetized:

1. Shave superficial fur from the neck and left side of the thorax using standard rodent clippers. Transfer the rat to a heating pad on a surgical board and secure in the supine recumbent position. Body temperature should be maintained at 37°C (± 1 °C)

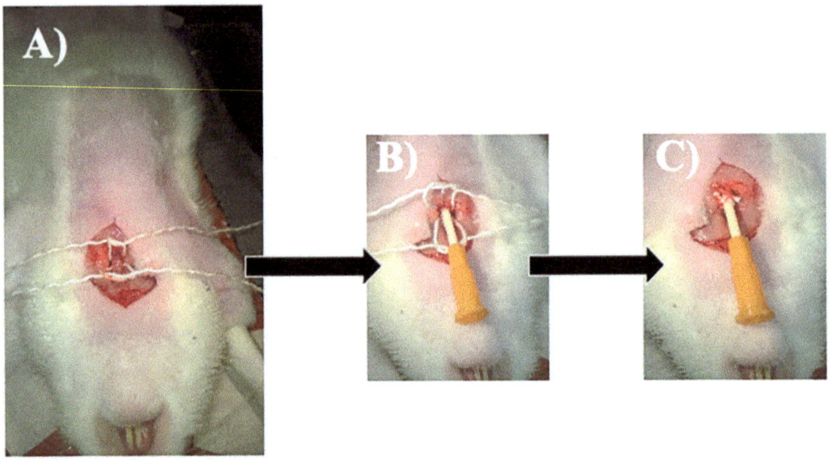

Fig. 1 Selected images demonstrating the tracheotomy procedure: (**a**) separation of sternohyoid muscles reveals the underlying trachea, allowing loose knots of ligature around the trachea prior to insertion of endotracheal cannula; (**b**) cannula inserted and advanced carefully; (**c**) ligature tightened, double knots formed to secure the cannula in place, and excess ligature cut

throughout the experiment using a rectal thermistor probe coupled with the thermostatically controlled heating pad.

2. *Tracheotomy*—In order to access the cardiac sympathetic nerve, a thoracotomy must be performed, which means the animal will need to be mechanically ventilated via a tracheal cannula. A vertical midline skin incision is made just below the jaw and extended to the sternum, followed by division and clearance of subcutaneous connective tissue using blunt dissection (Fig. 1a).
3. The sternohyoid muscles are separated to visualize the underlying trachea. Two strands of silk ligature (2–0) are loosely tied around the exposed tracheal segment, one rostrally and the other caudally, and a radial incision is made between two cartilaginous rings for the insertion of an endotracheal cannula (14 gauge angiocath) (Fig. 1b,c).
4. Finally, the trachea cannulated is connected to a rodent ventilator so that the animal can be mechanically ventilated: tidal volume ~ 1 mL/100 g BW and respiratory rate ~ 80–90-breaths/min. The inspirate gas is room air enriched with O_2.
5. *Thoracotomy*—Skin covering the left side of the thorax is removed (Fig. 2a), and the superficial pectoral fascia and the three pectoral muscle layers are removed using electrocautery to minimize blood loss. This exposes the underlying intercostal muscles and ribs (Fig. 2b).
6. Subsequently, the second, third, and fourth ribs are isolated and surgically removed by tying a ligature around the top

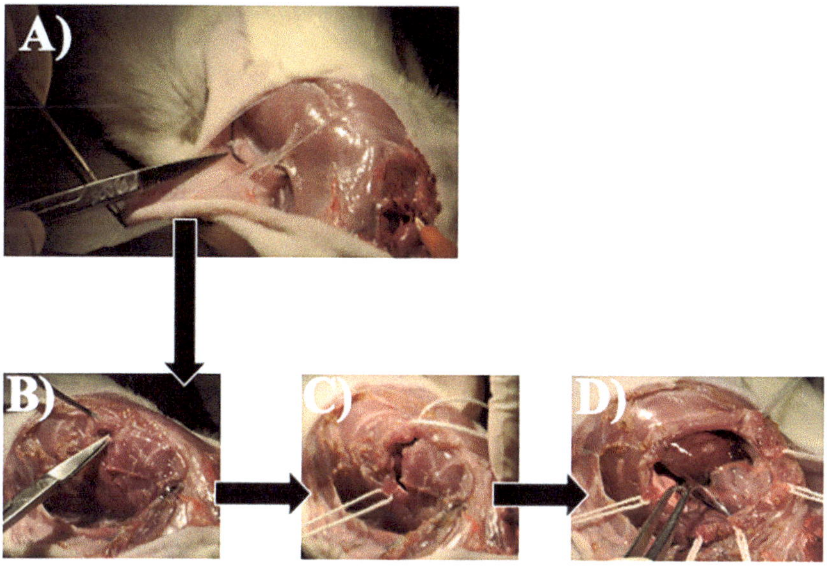

Fig. 2 Selected images illustrating the left thoracotomy procedure: (**a**) reflection of skin flap; (**b**) removal of pectoral muscle layers and blunt dissection through the intercostal muscle; (**c**) ligature tied at the medial and lateral region of the rib; (**d**) three ribs removed and ligature retracted radially to expose the heart and surrounding structures

(medial) and bottom (posterior) of each rib and then cutting out the segment of rib between the two ligature knots (Fig. 2c).

7. All ligatures that are tied to the ribs are retracted from the wound and securely taped to the surgical board, thereby generating a sufficient window for accessing the stellate ganglion (Fig. 2d), from which the cardiac sympathetic nerve arises [14].
8. *Isolation of the cardiac sympathetic nerve*—To enable visualization of the sympathetic trunk and stellate ganglion, the left lung must be gently retracted using soft saline-soaked cotton wool. (*see* **Note 5**)
9. Once the stellate ganglion is identified (Fig. 3a), the cardiac sympathetic nerve is confirmed (Fig. 3b) as the middle of three neural branches projecting medially from the stellate ganglion toward the heart. The nerve is very carefully dissected free from the surrounding tissue (Fig. 3c) using super-fine forceps and micro-scissors. Due to the frailty of the nerve, it is paramount to use extreme caution in order to prevent stretching or accidental touching of the nerve, as this greatly affects the viability of recorded electrical nerve signals [15].
10. The nerve is then sectioned ~5–6 mm distal to the stellate ganglion (Fig. 3d), and the proximal section (containing sympathetic efferent fibers) is carefully placed onto a pair of

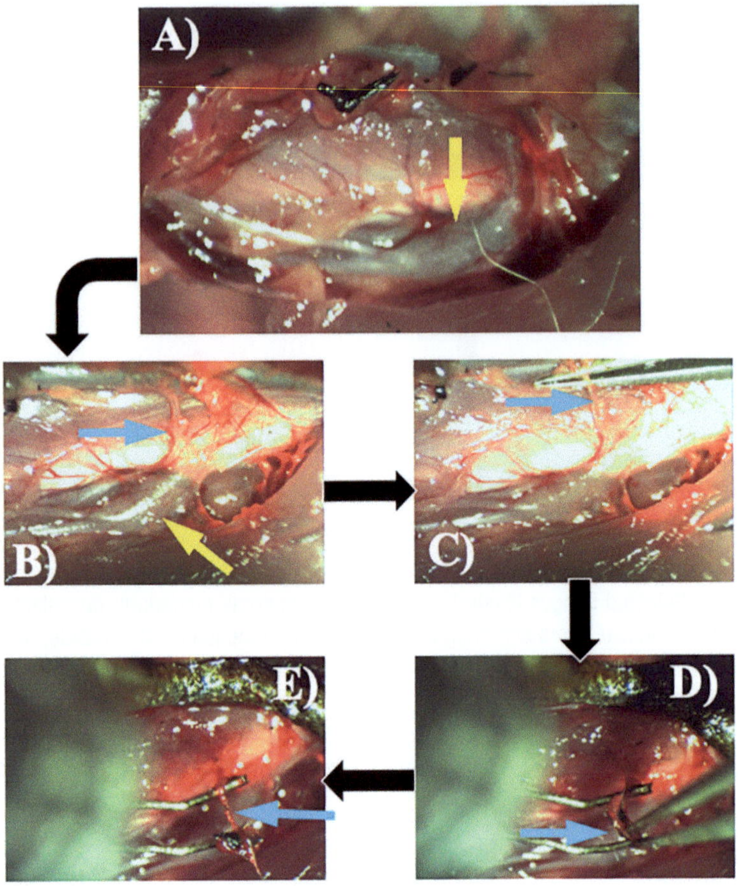

Fig. 3 Selected images showing the cardiac sympathetic nerve isolation procedure: (**a**) clearance of overlaying connective tissue to expose the stellate ganglion (yellow arrow); (**b**) cardiac sympathetic nerve identified (blue arrow); (**c**) nerve isolated from surrounding connective tissue. (**d**) nerve sectioned and further isolated from connective tissue. (**e**) platinum electrodes carefully lowered into position and nerve placed over, thereby enabling direct recording of cardiac SNA in real time

custom-made platinum recording electrodes using fine curved glass pipettes for handling the nerve (Fig. 3e) (*see* **Note 4**).

11. Once the nerve is on the electrode, the entire nerve/electrode preparation is covered with paraffin oil or silica gel to both insulate the nerve from surrounding electrical noise and interference, as well as prevent it from drying out and "dying" prematurely.
12. The animal preparation is now stable and the experimental protocol can commence.

3.2 Data Collection

Quantification of sympathetic nerve activity (SNA) using direct electrophysiological recordings is routine practice throughout the literature [16–19]. The method of quantifying the incoming raw new electroneurogram signal is described as follows:

1. The bipolar platinum electrodes are hardwired to a bio-amplifier that enhances and refines the incoming signal (Fig. 4a). An effective bio-amplifier should be capable of first filtering the incoming signal with a bandwidth filter between

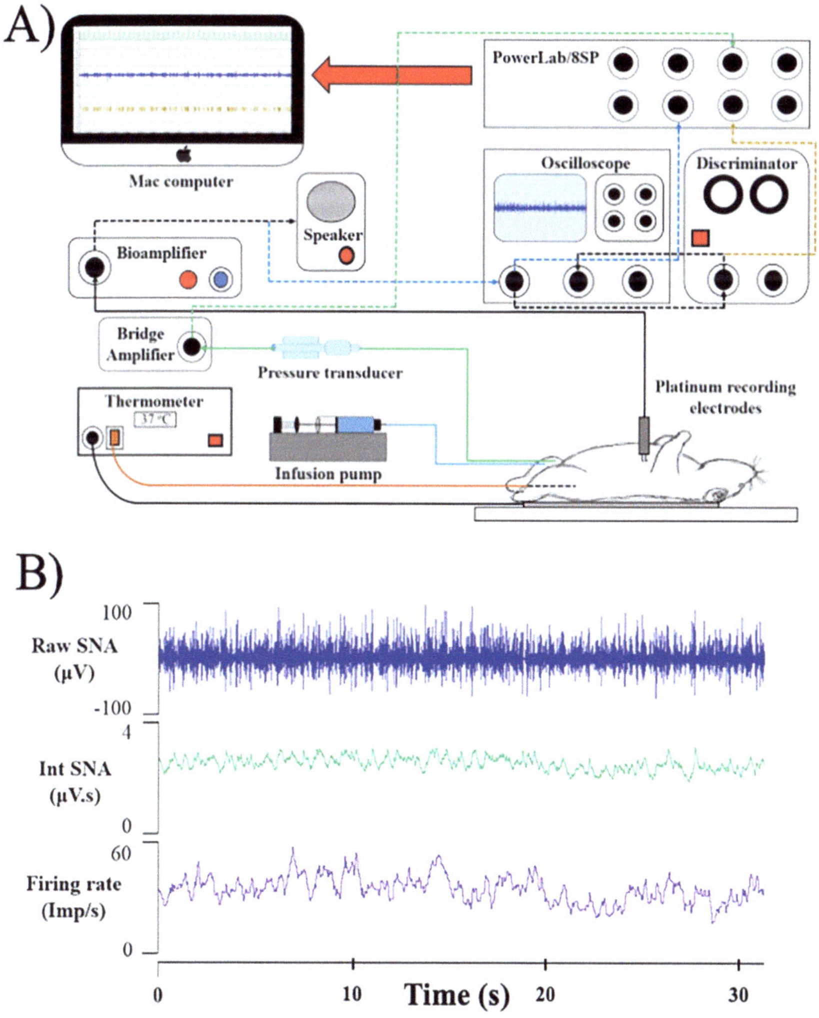

Fig. 4 (**a**) Schematic diagram of the equipment and experimental setup used for recording activity from the left cardiac sympathetic nerve in an anesthetized rat model. (**b**) Typical LabChart trace showing electrophysiological variables over time (30 s). From the raw SNA signal (blue), the inbuilt computational capabilities of the PowerLab data acquisition system allows instant calculation and display of integrated (Int) SNA (green) and firing rate (purple). SNA, sympathetic nerve activity; Int, integrated quantification of SNA in 10 s data bins; Imp/s, impulses per second

1 kHz (low-pass) and 0.1 kHz (high-pass). Second, the bio-amplifier should also be able to amplify a signal that is as small as 20 μV, by 10–25,000× .

2. Once the incoming neural signal has been filtered and amplified, it can then be relayed to an oscilloscope visualization of the real-time electrophysiological waveform (Fig. 4a).
3. Using a signal amplitude discriminator, the threshold for differentiating genuine nerve activity from electrical background noise can be set, thereby enabling the nerve firing rate to be derived from the raw signal. The presence of "clear" nerve activity can also assessed by an audio signal of the raw SNA, whereby "bursts" of SNA produce a distinct crackling sound against the background "white noise."
4. The signal can then be relayed from the bio-amplifier to a dedicated data acquisition system (e.g., PowerLab data acquisition system, AD Instruments), which is coupled with a PC computer. Importantly, the designated data acquisition system must have the capacity to continuously record SNA at a very high sampling rate (e.g., 4–10 kHz) in order to fully capture the entire temporal profile of action potential conduction along the nerve.
5. Quantification of the SNA signal is achieved by first rectifying the SNA signal and then integrating the rectified SNA signal. Signal quantification can be performed at pre-determined timed intervals so, for example, temporal changes in SNA over time can be observed. Moreover, the signal can also be dissected to tease out spike amplitude and spike frequency, which also provide simultaneous quantification of total nerve activity (Fig. 4b).

3.3 Equipment Calibration

The magnitude of the electroneurogram, associated with the propagation of action potentials along the sympathetic nerve, is in the order of microvolts (μV). In order to accurately quantify raw SNA the bio-amplifier needs to be calibrated. Our specific bio-amplifier (BMA-200 AC/DC, CWE Inc., USA) is equipped with an internal 100 μV calibration signal, which allows a two-point calibration (0 μV and 100 μV) to be performed, thereby providing an accurate measurement range of cardiac SNA [20].

3.4 Data Presentation: Absolute Versus Relative Change

The technique of recording cardiac sympathetic nerve activity (SNA) is associated with a high degree of data variability because, unlike a homeostatically controlled variable such as arterial blood pressure which is maintained at ~100 mmHg, there is no strictly defined or expected value for SNA. Rather, the value of SNA that is recorded from an isolated nerve preparation is dependent on multiple factors such as the following:

(i) The integrity or viability of the nerve preparation—remembering that the isolated nerve [bundle] contains multiple individual neural fibers so the total activity is the cumulative sum of activity of all fibers. However, during the surgical isolation of the nerve [bundle], some of the individual neural fibers are often damaged. Hence, variability in data can arise simply due to difference in the number of healthy individual neural fibers contributing to the overall electroneurogram between experiments.

(ii) The positioning of the nerve bundle on the recording electrodes. When the nerve is positioned on the two platinum recording electrodes, it is only those individual fibers that are either in direct contact or in close proximity to the electrode surface that will ultimately contribute to the electroneurogram. Therefore, variability in data can arise from difference in the number of individual neural fibers that are detected by the recording electrodes—which is dependent on positioning.

(iii) Inter-animal variation. Although a set-value is not expected for SNA, a narrow range of values can be attained if the surgical approach and experiment are repeated with a high degree of reproducibility—which can only be achieved through adequate training of personnel. In spite of the variability in SNA data within sample groups, one observable consistency for each recording is the magnitude of response, e.g., %increase following experimental intervention. Importantly, the magnitude of change following intervention should be considerably greater than the magnitude of variability within a sample population so that statistical analysis can still identify "significant" changes with somewhat small population sizes [16, 19, 21].

3.5 Conclusion

The electrophysiological recording of sympathetic nerve activity remains the gold-standard approach for accurately quantifying regional sympathetic traffic. However, surgical diligence and care are paramount to ensure a stable, reliable preparation that provides meaningful physiological data. Here, we are provided guidance on the approach and technique for specifically measuring cardiac sympathetic nerve activity in a laboratory rat model.

4 Notes

1. Urethane is supplied in a crystalline form, with which it must be dissolved in sterilized saline for a final concentration of 250 mg/ml. At such a high concentration, the solubility of urethane is relatively poor and so it is recommended that the

solution be heated (~40 °C) and stirred continuously for 10 min to enable urethane to be fully dissolved.

2. Platinum has exceptionally high electrical conductivity, is resistant to corrosion, is stable at high temperatures, and has stable electrical properties, making it an ideal material for electrophysiological recording of nerve activity. Two 10 mm strands of platinum wire (~0.3–0.4 mm in diameter) are soldered to the live and neutral strands of a standard three-strand electrical cable; the third "earth" lead is in direct contact with the animal (e.g., alligator clip) so as to ground the preparation and, thus, eliminate surrounding electrical interference. The platinum electrodes are shaped into two J-shaped hooks with which the nerve can be mounted.
3. Depending on the duration of the experimental protocol, sterilized saline can be administered to the animal preparation via a subcutaneous or intravenous injection, for the purpose of preserving fluid balance.
4. Placement of the platinum electrodes in the thorax cavity in close proximity to the isolated cardiac sympathetic nerve requires extreme caution so as to avoid any sudden movement that could bump and damage the nerve. Hence, it is recommended that a three-way axis micromanipulator that can move along the x, y, and z axis is used to slowly and carefully move the rod holding the bipolar electrode into position. This recommendation is based on 20 years of personal experience. No citation exists to reference this recommendation.
5. The size of the cardiac sympathetic nerve is almost impossible to visualize with the naked eye. Hence, a high-powered surgical microscope with 50–500× magnification and sufficient illumination is essential for the delicate surgical procedures described in this chapter.
6. Urethane is carcinogenic and so it is essential that appropriate PPE (mask and gloves) are used when preparing the urethane solution, and that the solution be prepared in a fume hood [13]. It is best to prepare a fresh batch of urethane solution each week.

References

1. May CN, Frithiof R, Hood SG, McAllen RM, McKinley MJ, Ramchandra R (2010) Specific control of sympathetic nerve activity to the mammalian heart and kidney. Exp Physiol 95: 34–40
2. Fechir M, Schlereth T, Kritzmann S, Balon S, Pfeifer N, Geber C, Breimhorst M, Eberle T, Gamer M, Birklein F (2009) Stress and thermoregulation: different sympathetic responses and different effects on experimental pain. Eur J Pain 13:935–941
3. Iriki M, Simon E (2012) Differential control of efferent sympathetic activity revisited. J Physiol Sci 62:275–298
4. Morrison SF (2001) Differential control of sympathetic outflow. Am J Physiol Regul Integr Comp Physiol 281:R683–R698

5. Lake CR, Major LF, Ziegler MG, Kopin IJ (1977) Increased sympathetic nervous system activity in alcoholic patients treated with disulfiram. Am J Psychiatry 134:1411–1414
6. Esler M, Kaye D (2000) Measurement of sympathetic nervous system activity in heart failure: the role of norepinephrine kinetics. Heart Fail Rev 5:17–25
7. Vaz M, Jennings G, Turner A, Cox H, Lambert G, Esler M (1997) Regional sympathetic nervous activity and oxygen consumption in obese normotensive human subjects. Circulation 96:3423–3429
8. Ishizawa T, Yoshiuchi K, Takimoto Y, Yamamoto Y, Akabayashi A (2008) Heart rate and blood pressure variability and baroreflex sensitivity in patients with anorexia nervosa. Psychosom Med 70:695–700
9. Nakamura Y, Yamamoto Y, Muraoka I (1993) Autonomic control of heart rate during physical exercise and fractal dimension of heart rate variability. J Appl Physiol (1985) 74:875–881
10. Kuwahara M, Yayou K, Ishii K, Hashimoto S, Tsubone H, Sugano S (1994) Power spectral analysis of heart rate variability as a new method for assessing autonomic activity in the rat. J Electrocardiol 27:333–337
11. Houle MS, Billman GE (1999) Low-frequency component of the heart rate variability spectrum: a poor marker of sympathetic activity. Am J Physiol 276:H215–H223
12. Arai Y, Saul JP, Albrecht P, Hartley LH, Lilly LS, Cohen RJ, Colucci WS (1989) Modulation of cardiac autonomic activity during and immediately after exercise. Am J Physiol 256:H132–H141
13. Maggi CA, Meli A (1986) Suitability of urethane anesthesia for physiopharmacological investigations in various systems. Part 2: Cardiovascular system. Experientia 42:292–297
14. Yasunaga K, Nosaka S (1979) Cardiac sympathetic nerves in rats: anatomical and functional features. Jpn J Physiol 29:691–705
15. Malpas SC (2010) Sympathetic nervous system overactivity and its role in the development of cardiovascular disease. Physiol Rev 90:513–557
16. Diong C, Jones PP, Tsuchimochi H, Gray EA, Hughes G, Inagaki T, Bussey CT, Fujii Y, Umetani K, Shirai M, Schwenke DO (2016) Sympathetic hyper-excitation in obesity and pulmonary hypertension: physiological relevance to the 'obesity paradox'. Int J Obes (Lond) 40:938–946
17. Hall TM, Gordon C, Roy R, Schwenke DO (2016) Delayed coronary reperfusion is ineffective at impeding the dynamic increase in cardiac efferent sympathetic nerve activity following myocardial ischemia. Basic Res Cardiol 111:35
18. Miki K, Kosho A, Hayashida Y (2002) Method for continuous measurements of renal sympathetic nerve activity and cardiovascular function during exercise in rats. Exp Physiol 87: 33–39
19. Roy RK, Augustine RA, Brown CH, Schwenke DO (2018) Activation of oxytocin neurons in the paraventricular nucleus drives cardiac sympathetic nerve activation following myocardial infarction in rats. Commun Biol 1:160
20. Thaung HP, Baldi JC, Wang HY, Hughes G, Cook RF, Bussey CT, Sheard PW, Bahn A, Jones PP, Schwenke DO, Lamberts RR (2015) Increased efferent cardiac sympathetic nerve activity and defective intrinsic heart rate regulation in type 2 diabetes. Diabetes 64: 2944–2956
21. Schwenke DO, Tokudome T, Kishimoto I, Horio T, Cragg PA, Shirai M, Kangawa K (2012) One dose of ghrelin prevents the acute and sustained increase in cardiac sympathetic tone after myocardial infarction. Endocrinology 153:2436–2443

Chapter 16

An Ovine Model of Chronic Heart Failure Induced by Repeated Coronary Microembolizations

Mridula Pachen and Rohit Ramchandra

Abstract

The use of large animals in research provides a unique bridge between preclinical findings and clinical relevance, offering a valuable perspective for advancing our understanding of the complexities of heart failure. Multiple models of heart failure have been established with advantages and limitations of each model. Many insights have been gained from these models for understanding both pathophysiological mechanisms and therapeutic interventions for heart failure. We have developed a chronic model of heart failure with reduced ejection fraction in sheep using the coronary microembolization technique. These animals gradually develop heart failure over a period of 3 months. In this chapter, we document how this model can be established. The left main coronary artery is cannulated under fluoroscopic guidance, and polystyrene latex microspheres are injected into the artery. Up to three sequential selective microembolizations are undertaken over a period of 3 weeks. Changes in ECG are monitored, and echocardiography is used to check on the progression of left ventricular dysfunction. All animals were followed for 3 months after the first embolization, and heart tissue was examined to check for changes in cardiac myocyte size. All animals developed stable signs of HF. We propose that multiple sequential intracoronary microembolizations can induce stable myocardial dysfunction with hemodynamic signs of chronic heart failure.

Key words Heart failure, Heart failure with reduced ejection fraction, Coronary microembolization, Coronary artery, Large animal model

1 Introduction

Heart failure with reduced ejection fraction (HFrEF) is associated with gradual deterioration of the left ventricular muscle, myocyte remodeling, and activation of autonomic and hormonal systems [1, 2]. Despite advancements in treatment and prevention, individuals with heart failure face a significant mortality rate [3] which remains unacceptably high. In this context, extensive research in both small and large animal models is pivotal in unraveling the pathogenesis of heart failure. While studies in rodent models of HFrEF have led to important advances, the development of clinically relevant large animal models of heart failure that can closely

Dhananjie N. K. Chandrasekera and Rajesh Katare (eds.), *Cardiomyocytes: Methods and Protocols*, Methods in Molecular Biology, vol. 2894, https://doi.org/10.1007/978-1-0716-4342-6_16,

mirror human heart failure is crucial to ensure that new treatments or paradigms can be tested in large animal models. Sheep, given their analogous heart anatomy and physiology to humans, provide a more accurate basis for comparing and studying HFrEF, and a number of different large animal models of heart failure have been developed and subsequently studied.

Animal models to mimic HFrEF include the pacing-induced model, doxorubicin infusion, coronary ligation, and coronary microembolization techniques. Pacing-induced HF [4–8] creates a consistent model of HFrEF with comparable hemodynamic and mechanical characteristics to human dilated cardiomyopathy. However, a drawback is the lack of tissue fibrosis if pacing is not prolonged. In addition, left ventricle dysfunction tends to reverse slowly upon termination of pacing, especially after short durations. Infusion of the cardiotoxin doxorubicin is another method that induces cardiac myocyte injury and HF [9]. However, its drawback includes inconsistent left ventricular dysfunction induction and lack of a reliable dosing strategy. While coronary ligation is more reflective of the clinical scenario, this model faces limitations as infarcts larger than 25% lead to increased left ventricular end-diastolic pressure and reduced stroke volume index, resulting in mortality rates exceeding 50%, often due to fatal arrhythmias or severe heart failure [10]. This is particularly true in sheep, where the anatomy can vary between animals, and this can lead to variable results. We have established the coronary microembolization model as a technique to induce chronic heart failure in sheep, where microspheres are injected into the coronary artery. The advantage of microembolization is that the model can be titrated to produce reproducible changes in heart function, and this chapter will lay out the methods for developing this model in sheep.

2 Materials

2.1 Animal Surgery

1. Before any animal experiments can be carried out, please make sure to ensure that the appropriate animal ethics approval has been received from the appropriate ethical governing body in your university/institution.
2. Adult sheep weighing 50–80 kg, housed in individual crates and acclimatized to laboratory conditions (we use the Romney cross females but Merino or other strains can also be used).
3. A surgical lab equipped with a mechanical ventilator and a patient table.
4. 2% Diprivan (propofol; 5 mg/kg IV).
5. 2% isoflurane–air–O_2 mixture.
6. Oxytetracycline (antibiotic; 6 mL).

7. Ketofen 10% (analgesia; 1 mL).
8. 18G Seldinger angiographic introducer needle.
9. 8Fr sheath introducer (CORDIS, USA).
10. 8F AL2 guide catheter (CORDIS, USA).
11. 0.035 × 150 cm PTFE angiography guide wire.
12. An X-ray angiography C-arm system (X-ray generators, imaging system, and workstation unit, Philips' Zenition Image-Mobile C-Arm System).
13. Iodine-based contrast materials.
14. Polystyrene latex microspheres.
15. β-Blocker (metoprolol up to 20 mg/kg, IV).
16. Lignocaine (2 mg/kg, IV).
17. Limb electrodes to record ECG.
18. Analog-to-digital recording set up (e.g., PowerLab and LabChart (ADInstruments, NZ)).
19. Hewlett Packard Sonos 1000 echocardiogram machine.

2.2 Masson's Trichrome Staining

1. Neutral buffered formalin.
2. 30% sucrose solution
3. Cryostat to section fixed ventricular tissue. 40 μm cryosection.
4. Bouin's solution: picric acid (supernatant); 75 mL.
5. 37–40% formaldehyde, 25 mL.
6. Glacial acetic acid, 5 mL.
7. Weigert's iron hematoxylin solution: stock solution A: 1 g hematoxylin, 95% alcohol, 100 mL; and stock solution B: 4 mL of 29% ferric chloride in water, 95 mL of distilled water, 1 mL of concentrated hydrochloric acid (*see* **Note 1**).
8. Biebrich scarlet–acid fuchsin solution: 1% aqueous Biebrich scarlet, 90 mL.
9. 1% aqueous acid fuchsin, 10 mL.
10. Glacial acetic acid, 1 mL.
11. 5% phosphotungstic acid/phosphomolybdic acid (PTA/PMA) solution: 5 gm phosphomolybdic acid, 100 mL distilled water.
12. Aniline blue solution: 2.5 g aniline blue, 2 mL glacial acetic acid, 100 mL distilled water.
13. 1% acetic acid solution: 1 mL glacial acetic acid, 99 mL distilled water.

3 Methods

1. The animal is given water access ad libitum but no access to food for the 24 h prior to induction of anesthesia.
2. The animal is coaxed into the crate, which allows access to the cephalic vein, and percutaneous access to this vein is obtained by experienced technicians.
3. Once access is confirmed with a saline flush, Diprivan is slowly injected into the vein to induce anesthesia in the animal. The depth of anesthesia is monitored closely to ensure that intubation can proceed.
4. The animal is then intubated using a pediatric endotracheal tube. This is also usually done by an experienced animal technician.
5. Following this, the animal is placed on a surgical table in a supine cradled position.
6. The right and left groin regions are shaved and cleaned using soap, followed by an antiseptic solution (Riodine® Povidone-Iodine antiseptic solution 10%). After thorough cleaning, both areas are further treated by spraying betadine solution.
7. Four needle electrodes are subcutaneously inserted into the left and right sides of the sternum and hind limbs, near the knee joint, for ECG recording. If needed, recordings are obtained from leads I, II, III, aVL, aVR, and aVF prior to the infusion of the microspheres and for a further 5 min after injection. Both lead I and lead II are the best leads for monitoring changes to the T-wave (*see* **Note 2**).
8. The recordings are made on a dual bio amp electrocardiograph switch box with PowerLab and LabChart.
9. Once baseline recordings of ECG have been established, percutaneous access to the left or right femoral artery is established using an 8F sheath. This is done by palpating the groin to visualize the arterial pulse and gaining access to the femoral artery using the Seldinger technique.
10. If blood analysis needs to be done, arterial blood samples (10 mL) can be collected into an EDTA vacutainer tube.
11. Following this, the AL2 guide catheter is filled with the contrast dye and then is inserted into the sheath and fed into the artery until the catheter is close to the heart under fluoroscopic guidance.
12. Under fluoroscopic guidance, the left main coronary artery is cannulated using the 8F AL2 guide catheter. The guide catheter is advanced till it reaches the base of the ascending aorta. Once the catheter is close to the heart, the catheter needs to be

gently rotated until it enters the left main coronary artery. The contrast dye is injected through the catheter into the coronary arteries to make the coronary vasculature visible on the X-ray images and confirm correct placement of the catheter.

13. The catheter can then be advanced into either the proximal left anterior descending (LAD) artery or left circumflex (LCX) artery if specific areas of embolization are required (*see* **Note 3**).
14. If needed, blood pressure can be monitored through the catheter by connecting it to the pressure tracing unit (*see* **Note 4**).
15. Upon securing the catheter position in the coronary artery, in preparation for polystyrene latex microsphere injection, an intravenous injection of β-blocker (metoprolol up to 20 mg/kg, IV) and lignocaine (2 mg/kg, IV) is administered to the venous line in the forelimb, to prevent ventricular arrhythmias.
16. Once the drugs are injected, 1.2–1.4 mL of microspheres are injected into the coronary artery (*see* **Note 5**). ECG recordings are closely monitored throughout the procedure. A change in the ST segment (elevation or depression) and T-wave (inversion) on one or more limb leads should be observed within minutes of the injection. This can be taken as an indication of successful embolization (*see* **Note 6** and Fig. 1).
17. At the end of the procedure, the antibiotic oxytetracycline (6 mL) is given intramuscularly. In addition, the analgesic Ketofen (10%; 1 mL) is also given intramuscularly.
18. The animal is recovered from the anesthetic and following recovery, moved into the crate or pen (*see* **Note 7**).
19. Echocardiograms are obtained at the end of 1 week of first embolization to confirm ejection fraction (EF). Ejection fraction was obtained in the long-axis and short-axis M-mode views (*see* **Note 8**).
20. If the ejection fraction is still high (over 55%), then a second embolization is done. These embolizations are spaced 1 week apart and we have undertaken up to a maximum of three embolizations in each animal.
21. Echocardiography can be used to monitor the decline in left ventricular function throughout the months after the embolization. In our hands, the animals have a consistent depressed ejection fraction after the first embolization with some variability between animals. We leave the animals for around 2–-3 months to ensure fibrosis is present and allows us to experiment with a *chronic* model of heart failure.

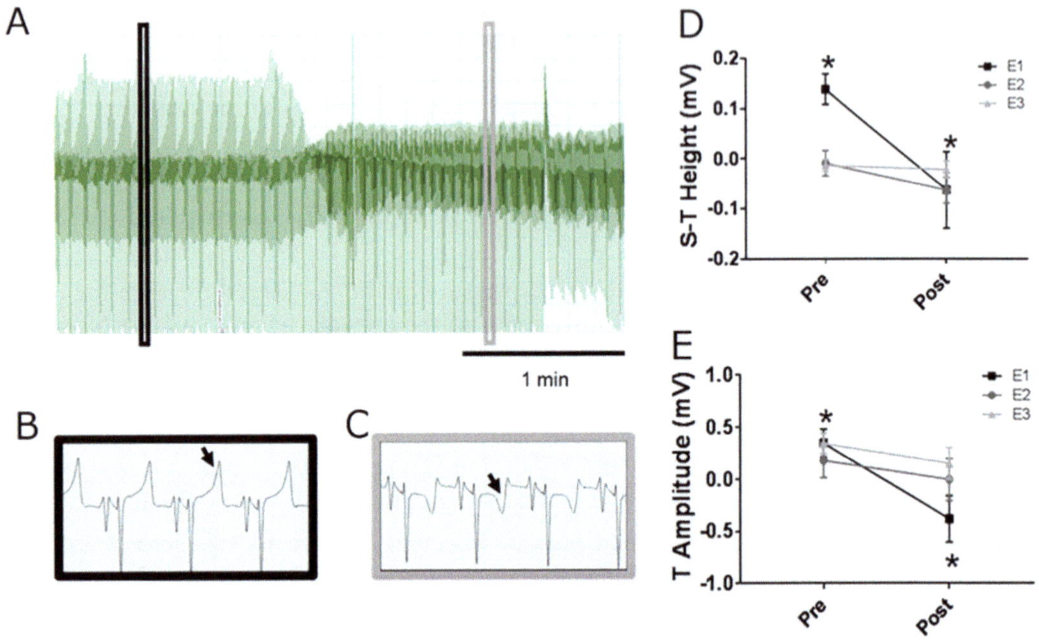

Fig. 1 Representative electrocardiogram traces in sheep before and after microembolizations and mean data on S–T and T-wave segments. (**a**) Lead II trace highlighting the changes over time in the ECG, with (**b**) highlighting magnified lead II activity before microembolization and (**c**) after microembolization. Arrows highlight the T-wave of the ECG, showing a depression after microembolization. (**d**) Mean data on the height of the S–T segment and (**e**) T-wave amplitude before and after the individual microembolization procedures. Pre- indicates before microembolization and post- after microembolization. Microembolization 1 (E1) represented by square, microembolization 2 (E2) by circle, and microembolization 3 (E3) by triangle. (*$p < 0.05$ in E1 only, $n = 6$). (Figure taken from [11])

3.1 Cardiac Collagen Tissue Collection and Measurement

1. Hearts were collected at the end of the experiment and a portion of the left ventricle free wall can be fixed in neutral buffered formalin.
2. Following 24 h for fixing of the tissue, the tissue blocks are transferred to a 30% sucrose solution for preservation.
3. Following at least 48 h, the heart blocks are cut into 40 μm sections using a cryostat to allow for staining of tissue.
4. To measure collagen deposition, sections of the hearts are stained with Masson's trichrome stain (MTS) solution. In Masson's trichrome staining, cardiac muscle fibers typically stain red, while collagen stains blue (Fig. 2).
5. Following the staining, sections are subjected to two washes with distilled water and then three changes of 100% ethanol.
6. Finally, a final wash is undertaken with xylene solution before cover slipping.

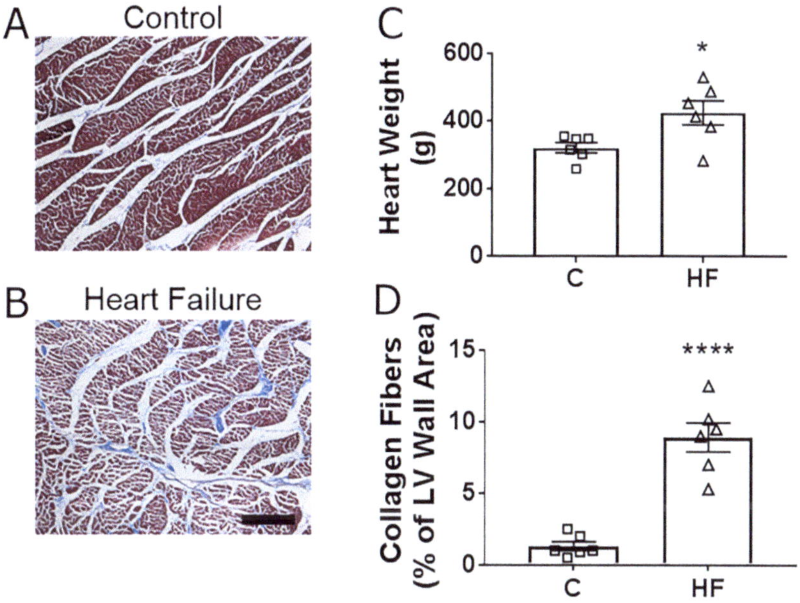

Fig. 2 Representative sheep cardiac tissue images and effect of microembolizations on collagen deposition and heart weight. (**a**) shows section of the left ventricle wall from a sheep heart in a control healthy animal (HF) and (**b**) shows section of the left ventricle wall in a sheep with heart failure, taken 16 weeks after microembolization. (**c**) Heart weights of both control (represented by squares) and heart failure (represented by triangles) sheep. (**d**) illustrates the collagen content in control and heart failure sheep, $^{*}p < 0.05$, $^{****}p < 0.0001$. Bars represent mean values ± SEM. Data from individual sheep are illustrated with symbols. *C* control (square), *HF* (triangle), *LV* left ventricle of heart. Scale bar = 100 μm. (Figure taken from [11])

4 Notes

1. Mix equal parts of stock solutions A and B to make up fresh Weigert's iron hematoxylin working solution each time.
2. Recording of ECG in sheep necessitates good contact with electrodes and we have used needles soldered to the ECG wires. While ECG electrodes usually come with sticky patch electrodes, the lanolin on the skin means that these electrodes tend to not work as well as needle electrodes.
3. Catheter cannulation process is very similar to a coronary angiogram procedure. Care must be taken not to tear or damage the coronary arteries. It is advisable to seek assistance from an interventional cardiologist to ensure the procedure is conducted safely and effectively. Also note that the origin of the coronary artery when entering through the left ventricle may be different due to differing anatomy in different animals. Sometimes it may be useful to use a different access catheter with a slightly different angle depending on the animal anatomy.

4. If the blood pressure trace looks inconsistent, ensure that the catheter is not wedged around the artery. If either of these situations is observed, gently pull back the catheter without unhooking (removing) it from the coronary artery until a clean and smooth waveform is visible.
5. The microspheres are stored at −20 °C but need to be warmed up to ensure that the spheres do not clump together. We usually warm them in hand and constantly shake them for around 5 min before injecting them into the coronary arteries. In earlier experiments, we found that occasionally we do not get ECG changes which may reflect that the microspheres do not disperse as well. Also note that depending on the area that is embolized, the ECG pattern may be altered preferentially in one of the leads. We find that if no change is detected, then altering to a different lead usually reveals a change in the ECG.
6. The ECG changes tend to be most prominent for the first embolization. In subsequent embolizations, there should still be a change in the T-wave, although the extent of the change is usually less than the first one.
7. Blood pressure tends to decrease after the embolization, so careful monitoring of the animal is needed post the embolization. Occasionally, if the embolization is severe, the animal may experience congestion and labored breathing. In this scenario, we give furosemide intravenously to help with decongestion. In some cases, we need to give multiple doses of furosemide to improve the condition of the animal.
8. A human echocardiographic machine with an adult transthoracic probe was used in all our studies but different probes can be trialed.

Acknowledgements

This work was supported by grants to RR from the Health Research Council of New Zealand, the National Heart Foundation of New Zealand, and the University of Auckland Faculty Research Development Fund.

References

1. Jackson G, Gibbs C, Davies M, Lip G (2000) ABC of heart failure: pathophysiology. Br Med J 320(7228):167
2. Kemp CD, Conte JV (2012) The pathophysiology of heart failure. Cardiovasc Pathol 21(5): 365–371
3. Falk V, Garbade J, Walther T (2005) Experimental models of heart failure. In: Practical methods in cardiovascular research. Springer, pp 83–110
4. Timek TA, Dagum P, Lai DT, Liang D, Daughters GT, Tibayan F et al (2003) Tachycardia-induced cardiomyopathy in the ovine heart: mitral annular dynamic

three-dimensional geometry. J Thorac Cardiovasc Surg 125(2):315–324

5. Byrne MJ, Kaye DM, Mathis M, Reuter DG, Alferness CA, Power JM (2004) Percutaneous mitral annular reduction provides continued benefit in an ovine model of dilated cardiomyopathy. Circulation 110(19):3088–3092
6. Ramchandra R, Xing DT, Matear M, Lambert G, Allen AM, May CN (2019) Neurohumoral interactions contributing to renal vasoconstriction and decreased renal blood flow in heart failure. Am J Phys Regul Integr Comp Phys 317(3):R386–RR96
7. Ramchandra R, Hood SG, Denton DA, Woods RL, McKinley MJ, McAllen RM et al (2009) Basis for the preferential activation of cardiac sympathetic nerve activity in heart failure. Proc Natl Acad Sci 106(3):924–928
8. Ramchandra R, Hood S, Xing D, Lambert G, May C (2018) Mechanisms underlying the increased cardiac norepinephrine spillover in heart failure. Am J Physiol Heart Circ Physiol 315:H340
9. Borenstein N, Bruneval P, Behr L, Laborde F, Montarras D, Daurès JP et al (2006) An ovine model of chronic heart failure: echocardiographic and tissue Doppler imaging characterization. J Card Surg 21(1):50–56
10. Hood WB Jr, McCarthy B, LOWN B. (1967) Myocardial infarction following coronary ligation in dogs: hemodynamic effects of isoproterenol and acetylstrophanthidin. Circ Res 21(2):191–200
11. Abukar Y, Lever N, Pachen M, LeGrice IJ, Ramchandra R (2019) Impaired baroreflex function in an ovine model of chronic heart failure induced by multiple coronary microembolizations. Front Physiol 10:1420

Index

Dhananjie N. K. Chandrasekera and Rajesh Katare (eds.), *Cardiomyocytes: Methods and Protocols*, Methods in Molecular Biology, vol. 2894, https://doi.org/10.1007/978-1-0716-4342-6,

M

N

O

P

Q

R

S

T

V

W

MIX
Papier aus verantwortungsvollen Quellen
Paper from responsible sources
FSC® C105338

If you have any concerns about our products,
you can contact us on
ProductSafety@springernature.com

In case Publisher is established outside the EU,
the EU authorized representative is:
Springer Nature Customer Service Center GmbH
Europaplatz 3, 69115 Heidelberg, Germany

Printed by Libri Plureos GmbH
in Hamburg, Germany